PSYCH - LITE

Notice

Medicine is an ever-changing science. As new research and clinical experience broaden our knowledge, changes in treatment and drug therapy are required. The editors and the publisher of this work have checked with sources believed to be reliable in their efforts to provide information that is complete and generally in accord with the standards accepted at the time of publication. However, in view of the possibility of human error or changes in medical sciences, neither the editors, nor the publisher, nor any other party who has been involved in the preparation or publication of this work warrants that the information contained herein is in every respect accurate or complete. Readers are encouraged to confirm the information contained herein with other sources. For example, and in particular, readers are advised to check the product information sheet included in the package of each drug they plan to administer to be certain that the information contained in this book is accurate and that changes have not been made in the recommended dose or in the contraindications for administration. This recommendation is of particular importance in connection with new or infrequently used drugs.

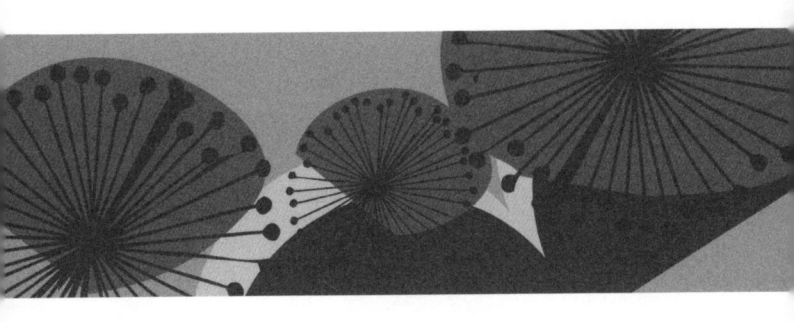

PSYCH - LITE
PSYCHIATRY THAT'S EASY TO READ

ROB SELZER & STEVE ELLEN

The McGraw·Hill Companies

Sydney New York San Francisco Auckland
Bangkok Bogotá Caracas Hong Kong
Kuala Lumpur Lisbon London Madrid
Mexico City Milan New Delhi San Juan
Seoul Singapore Taipei Toronto

Copyright © 2010 McGraw-Hill Australia Pty Limited
Additional owners of copyright are acknowledged in on-page credits.

Every effort has been made to trace and acknowledge copyrighted material. The authors and publishers tender their apologies should any infringement have occurred.

Reproduction and communication for educational purposes
The Australian *Copyright Act 1968* (the Act) allows a maximum of one chapter or 10% of the pages of this work, whichever is the greater, to be reproduced and/or communicated by any educational institution for its educational purposes provided that the institution (or the body that administers it) has sent a Statutory Educational notice to Copyright Agency Limited (CAL) and been granted a licence. For details of statutory educational and other copyright licences contact: Copyright Agency Limited, Level 15, 233 Castlereagh Street, Sydney NSW 2000. Telephone: (02) 9394 7600. Website: www.copyright.com.au

Reproduction and communication for other purposes
Apart from any fair dealing for the purposes of study, research, criticism or review, as permitted under the Act, no part of this publication may be reproduced, distributed or transmitted in any form or by any means, or stored in a database or retrieval system, without the written permission of McGraw-Hill Australia including, but not limited to, any network or other electronic storage.

Enquiries should be made to the publisher via www.mcgraw-hill.com.au or marked for the attention of the permissions editor at the address below.

National Library of Australia Cataloguing-in-Publication Data	
Author:	Selzer, Robert.
Title:	Psych-lite : psychiatry that's easy to read / Robert Selzer, Steven Ellen.
Edition:	1st ed.
ISBN:	9780070998001 (pbk.)
Notes:	Includes index.
Subjects:	Psychiatry–Textbooks.
Other Authors/Contributors:	Ellen, Steven.
Dewey Number:	616.89

Published in Australia by
McGraw-Hill Australia Pty Ltd
Level 2, 82 Waterloo Road, North Ryde NSW 2113
Publisher: Elizabeth Walton
Editorial coordinator: Fiona Richardson
Art director: Astred Hicks
Cover design and illustration: Damien Matter
Internal design: Simon Rattray, Squirt Creative
Production editor: Emel Gusic
Copy editor: Marcia Bascombe
Proofreader: Leila Jabbour
Indexer: Michael Ramsden
Typeset in India by Mukesh Technologies
Printed in China by iBook Printing Ltd on 100gsm woodfree

~ Dedication ~

We thought long and hard about who most influenced the way we think and teach.

It's our fathers, Paul and Cliff, to whom we dedicate this book.

Foreword

Rob was a born communicator (says Steve) and Steve doesn't teach so much as entertain (says Rob) in their respective 'biopics' for this little book. They point out that it is intentionally oversimplistic and not enough to pass exams, but intended to help the student hit the road running.

In *Psych-Lite*, Rob and Steve, both clinical academics at Monash University and the Alfred Hospital, have prepared the almost perfect appetiser. Their serious but irreverent approach to teaching is demonstrated by their liberal use of mnemonics to help the student remember key points. It is full of little gems, summarising topics that normally occupy whole chapters or books in less than a thousand words. Perhaps my favourite is the chapter on formulation with its wonderful table of prompts—I am sure many a psychiatry registrar will wish they had this to hand when it came to preparing for the dreaded clinical long case.

Like any good appetiser, *Psych-Lite* will leave any student with more than a passing interest in psychiatry, whether literal or metaphorical, hungry for more. Although the book has been written for medical students, it is the sort of quick reference guide that could usefully grace the shelves, or preferably the desks, of general practitioners and many allied health professionals.

Robert Adler
Psychiatrist, Melbourne

CONTENTS

Foreword vii
Contents ix
Preface xi
About the authors xii
Acknowledgments xiv

1 Classification: the secret key to understanding psychiatry 1
2 Taking a history 7
3 Mental state examination 12
4 Making a diagnosis: proposing a formulation 18
5 Risk assessment 23
6 Mood disorders 29
7 Schizophrenia 35
8 Anxiety disorders 40
9 Drug and alcohol disorders 46
10 Personality disorders 52
11 Consultation-liaison psychiatry 57
12 Medications 62
13 Psychotherapies 69
14 Child and adolescent psychiatry 74
15 Old age psychiatry 79

Index 85

Preface

The purpose of *Psych-lite* is to give you the essence of psychiatry, as needed by medical students. We've tried to make *Psych-lite* brief, enjoyable and very practical. The text is written in plain English, and each chapter has been deliberately restricted to less than 1000 words.

Psych-lite is deliberately non-comprehensive. We haven't covered all the major illnesses or covered any in depth. But we have described some of the types of disorders that you need to be familiar with as medical students. The descriptions are enough to give you an overview but you'll need to do more reading. The idea is to provide just enough knowledge so that you'll know what you need to know. This book alone is not enough to pass exams or even write up case histories (not by a long shot), but it will help you hit the road running when you start your rotation.

Psych-lite is intentionally over-simplistic. A lot of the concepts in psychiatry can be complex, controversial and difficult to understand. We reckon to grasp the complexities, it's easier if you start from a simple base. From there you can learn the exceptions, nuances and controversies: *simple first, complex later*. But this does mean that you'll need to learn topics in more depth, i.e. don't stop your psychiatry reading here.

Rob Selzer and Steve Ellen

About the authors

Rob Selzer (written by Steve):
Rob was a born communicator. Back in school, he told us a mnemonic he developed to remember the prices in the tuck shop. Did you know a sausage roll cost only 35 cents back then? (This was before Rob turned vegetarian.) Anyway, since then he's continued his passion—and done pretty much all the degrees a doctor can do. Now an associate professor, he's in charge of medical student teaching at Alfred Health and undergraduate psychiatry teaching at Monash Uni. Rob loves thinking outside the square, injecting life into teaching programs and enthusing others to teach and to learn.

Rob genuinely believes his children are gifted and are the reason the world was created (obviously he hasn't met my son). He is a true good guy—yoga, the environment, family and friends... I think you get the picture. He co-created and still hosts one of Melbourne's oldest medical chat shows on radio (I think it's clocked up about 15 years). If I were to sum him up—he's a guy who loves hearing new ideas and breathing life into them (oh, and he loves chatting to everyone too). This book was Rob's idea, and I thank him for bringing me on board.

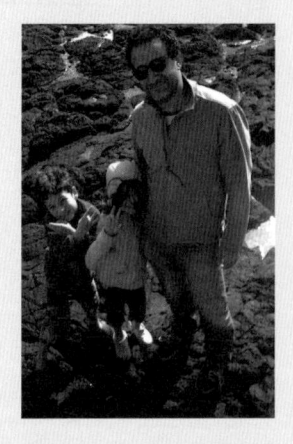

Rob is third from the left

Steve Ellen (written by Rob):

When I met Steve in high school I came away thinking, 'This guy wants to be a doctor, but he wants to be everything else as well'. Back then I thought it was a little optimistic, but I wasn't far off the mark—Steve has represented Australia in triathlon (Masters), plays drums in a band and he's an associate professor in psychiatry.

I just deleted a long list of some of the things he's done along the way because it went way over our word limit— let's just say he's an exceptionally accomplished clinician and leader. He now heads the consultation, liaison and emergency psychiatry unit at Alfred Health and is respected both within and outside of the profession.

Watching Steve take a tute or give a lecture is always an adventure. He doesn't teach so much as entertain. Through his good humour, enthusiasm and compassion, his audience learns. Steve's motto is 'Education can fix pretty much everything'. Writing with him was a whole other adventure!

(Yep, I know his son, Billy, and I can see why Steve thinks the world was created too.)

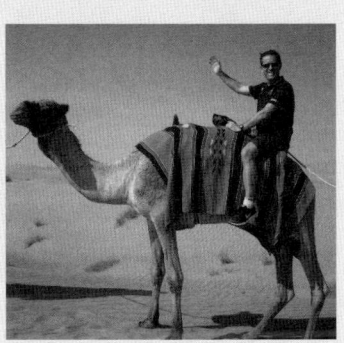

Steve is the one waving

Acknowledgments

Dr James Nahamkes provided us with advice and criticism, some of it about the book's contents. Our students supplied us with an almost endless list of creative questions and shaped our ideas on teaching psychiatry. Our patients over the years have taught us many lessons you just can't get from books. For putting up with us, our publisher, Elizabeth Walton and editorial coordinator Fiona Richardson from McGraw-Hill, deserve more than words. We are also indebted to our many colleagues and friends who offered us guidance and support.

1

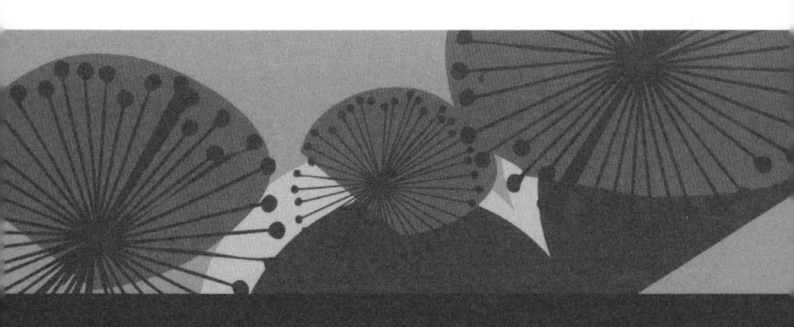

Classification: the secret key to understanding psychiatry

This is probably the chapter you are going to want to skip. You can if you want to but if you know what's in this chapter, then the rest of psychiatry will be much easier to understand. It's a 'stitch in time saves nine' type of chapter. If you understand classification, you will understand psychiatry.

IMPORTANCE OF CLASSIFICATION

Classification underpins what gets called 'mental illness'. If someone has a 'mental illness', then they require treatment. Unlike physical symptoms, where everyone understands that pain or fever or some other symptom means *visit the doctor*, in psychiatry it is not so simple. If you get anxious do you get help? If you are one of the few people who do, do you go to friends, family, the publican, a minister of religion, a psychologist or a doctor? Classification defines what we as a group of doctors think. It says *these are illnesses, and if you get them please visit us*! As you will see, classification in psychiatry is not as simple as in physical medicine (e.g. pain or fever).

> *Psychiatrists focus on complaints that appear in people's thoughts, perception, moods and behaviours, rather than skin, bones, muscles, and viscera.* – McHugh & Slavney[1]

DISTINGUISHING NORMAL FROM ABNORMAL

What is normal? Go on, try to define 'normal'. Difficult, isn't it? But we're psychiatrists so we need to at least try.

For a given symptom, how do you define the cut-off point? How depressed do you have to be to have a depressive disorder? When does fear of a spider become a phobia? When does a wacky idea become a delusion? Just because Rob and Steve believe they are going to win a Nobel prize, does that mean they are delusional?

To get around the problem of separating normal from abnormal, we do a few things. First we find associated symptoms that go together to form a 'syndrome'. Then we arbitrarily define a cut-off point based on the number of symptoms. Next, we usually insist on a minimum time frame. Finally, there must be either severe distress or interference with functioning for the diagnosis of disorder to be made. So for depression, you have to have five of nine symptoms, for at least two weeks, causing clinically significant distress or impairment in social, occupational or other important areas of functioning (from the *Diagnostic and Statistical Manual of Mental Disorders*[2]). Thus, 'abnormal' is separated from 'normal'.

Most syndromes, diseases (a syndrome with an organic basis) and disorders (somewhere between a disease and a syndrome) are best thought of as dimensions, as there is a smooth or continuous transition from normal to abnormal. But for the sake of simplicity, they are described and communicated as categories (separate entities in their own right).

THE DIAGNOSTIC HIERARCHY

Having established the ground rules for distinguishing normal from abnormal, the next principle that guides classification is the *diagnostic hierarchy*. This is a hierarchy of the key psychiatric disorders, whereby the disorder highest

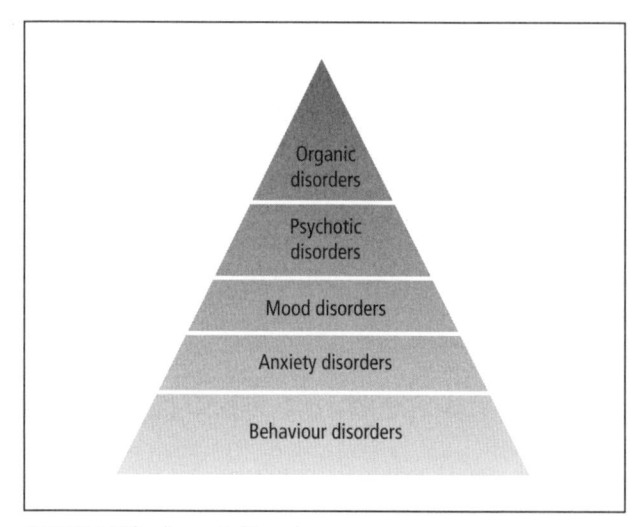

FIGURE 1.1 The diagnostic hierarchy

on the hierarchy takes diagnostic precedence over those below. Put another way, disorders higher on the hierarchy can cause all the symptoms below on the hierarchy as well as their own.

If a patient has an organic disorder, they will have symptoms of either memory problems or decreased consciousness, or other symptoms such as psychotic symptoms or mood symptoms. If the patient presents with a psychotic disorder, they will have psychotic symptoms, plus mood, anxiety or behaviour symptoms, but they should *not* have organic symptoms. If they have a mood disorder, they can have mood symptoms and those below, but *not* organic or psychotic symptoms. (The exception here is the affective psychoses.) In anxiety disorders, expect anxiety and behaviour symptoms, but *not* mood, psychotic or organic symptoms. Behaviour disorders can only have behaviour symptoms.

When making a diagnosis, we think of all the patient's symptoms, and the symptoms highest on the hierarchy give the most likely diagnosis. So if a person presents with depression, some anxiety symptoms and hallucinations, but has no memory impairment or decreased conscious state, the most likely diagnosis is schizophrenia.

You must also consider the timeline of symptoms. If a patient presents with a history of two years of anxiety and depression, but nothing above on the hierarchy, we will diagnose depression, as it accounts for all the symptoms. If, however, they have had the anxiety symptoms for two years but the depressed mood for six months, we might consider that the patient has had an anxiety disorder for two years, and then developed comorbid depression six months ago.

DIAGNOSTIC MANUALS

These two basic principles—the differentiation of normal from abnormal and the diagnostic hierarchy—form the basis of our classification systems. As you might imagine, the classifications change over time. This is partly because we learn more about the symptoms and disorders, but also because society changes its views about symptoms and disorders. For example, in the 1960s homosexuality was considered abnormal behaviour and was in the diagnostic manuals. More recently, gambling has been considered an abnormal behaviour in some extreme circumstances and so has entered the diagnostic manuals. Disorders go in and out of style according to knowledge, research and societal beliefs.

The most popular manual in psychiatry (in the USA and Australia) is the *Diagnostic and Statistical Manual of Mental Disorders* produced by the American Psychiatric Association (called DSM or DSM-IV, referring to the fourth edition for short). It uses the basic principles above. The DSM was the catalyst for most of the modern classification work in psychiatry.

References

1 McHugh, PR & Slavney, PR 1986, *The Perspectives of Psychiatry*, John Hopkins University Press, Baltimore Maryland.

2 American Psychiatric Association 1994, *Diagnostic and Statistical Manual of Mental Disorders*, 4th edn, American Psychiatric Association, Washington DC.

2

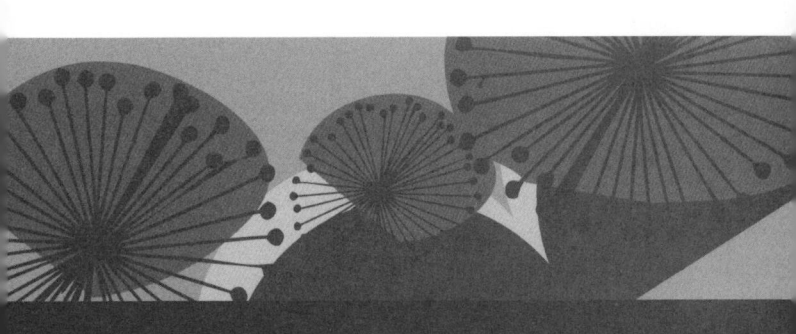

Taking a history

You have three goals when taking a history at assessment (i.e. interviewing a new patient):

1. Make a diagnosis (repeat this goal to yourself twice now—it's important but often lost during the interview process)
2. Build a formulation (an explanation of the patient's presentation)
3. Form a trusting, therapeutic relationship with the patient.

HOW TO TAKE A HISTORY

Start by asking the patient something not emotionally charged, such as their demographic details. Next, ask what medication has been prescribed. The medication list gives you an idea of what other doctors think the diagnosis might be. Next, ask what brought the patient to hospital:

Tell me a little about what brings you here today?

At this point, allow the patient to talk uninterrupted for about five minutes—free talk. Free talk is important for three reasons. Firstly, it allows the patient to feel heard. This is one of the most important parts of the patient–doctor relationship. Secondly, it allows you to detect any formal thought disorder (illogical patterns of thinking—we'll discuss this again in mental state examination later). This is easily missed if you proceed down a 'tennis match' of a question-answer pattern. Thirdly, it lets information out so you can see which way the diagnosis is heading. In psychiatry it would be impossible to make a diagnosis without some sort of a lead. If you don't allow the patient to free talk at the start then you don't have a lead.

Now, at the end of five minutes you should have an idea as to where you think the main problem lies. This will be a hypothesis, so you proceed down that path until you are convinced you're on the right track or you reckon you should try another path. The trick is to try one path at a time rather than try all tracks at once.

Below is a list of some of the main problems in patients who present to psychiatrists.

- Mood disorders
- Psychosis
- Personality disorder
- Adjustment disorder
- Anxiety disorders—OCD, PTSD, GAD, SAD, PA, PD
- Drug and alcohol disorders
- Delirium
- Dementia
- Somatic disorders
- Life issues, such as grief, loss, divorce

After the first five minutes pick one of these areas and see if it fits the patient presentation. You can start by using a screening question. Here are some of the screening questions we use to elicit disorders that may not be readily apparent (think of this as an equivalent to a systems review in medicine).

Anxiety disorders
Obsessive compulsive disorder
Do you find that you need to check things many times or perform little 'rituals' so something bad won't happen?

Post-traumatic stress disorder
Some people who have had a traumatic event in their life can relive it over and over, and avoid anything that reminds them of the event. Has that happened to you?

Panic disorder/panic attacks
Have you ever had a panic attack?

Social anxiety disorder
Do you miss social engagements out of fear that people may not like you or that they might think poorly of you?

Generalised anxiety disorder
Do you worry a lot ... about little day-to-day things that you just can't seem to get off your mind?

Depression
Over the last couple of weeks has your mood been down most of the time? Or have you not enjoyed things that you would normally enjoy?

Bipolar disorder
(screen for mania)

Have you ever felt extra good or too good?

Or

Have you had a period of time where you didn't need to sleep much and you did impulsive things, or things out of character?

Psychosis
Have you had any unusual experiences lately?
Have you heard voices or sounds when no-one else has been in the room?

Do you get a sense that someone or some people mean you harm?

Now, remember that these are screening questions. If the patient answers 'yes' it doesn't automatically mean they have the disorder. It means you need to investigate more.

By the end of the interview you should have an idea of what the possible diagnoses may be. Your mental state exam should add evidence to your diagnosis. The key (just like in medicine) is to make a diagnosis based on reliable information and then make a corresponding management plan.

Sometimes psychiatric diagnoses are not easy to make following an assessment interview, so psychiatrists make a provisional diagnosis and then list differential diagnoses as well. You should do this for all patients you assess too. It ensures that you don't have 'premature closure' (i.e. sticking to one diagnosis even if new, contrary information comes to hand). In psychiatry there is very often more information to be gleaned that can either confirm or refute your provisional diagnosis.

Don't forget you also need to enquire into:

- activities of daily living (ADLs) such as self-care, household chores and grocery shopping
- past psychiatric history
- forensic history
- past medical history
- family history, including family functioning
- developmental history
- personality—ask a question such as:

How would someone who knows you well describe you? How would you describe yourself? How do you cope with stressful situations?

3

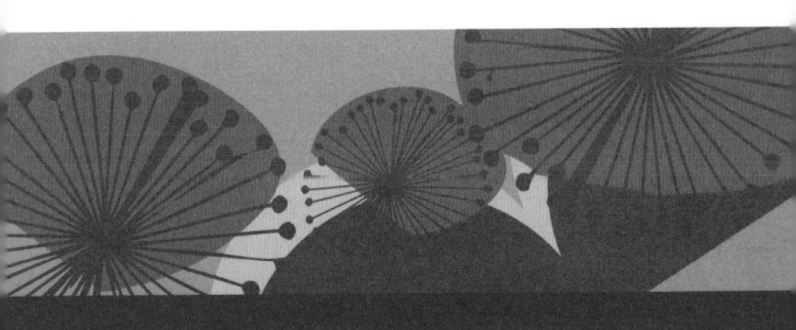

Mental state examination

Ophthalmologists have ophthalmoscopes, neurologists have plessors and psychiatrists have the mental state examination (MSE). The MSE is the 'objective' examination the psychiatrist performs. It is objective in that it relies on direct observation as distinct from the history, which relies on the patient's subjective description.

THE MSE
Some patients will require more description in a particular area of the mental state examination than other areas. For example, for a patient with psychosis you should include a lot of information about thought form. Below are the main areas of the MSE.

Appearance
Imagine you have a photograph of the patient. Describe what you see.

Clothing Dishevelled clothing could indicate the patient is disorganised as occurs in schizophrenia or uncaring about appearance as happens in depression. Bright or overly revealing clothes could indicate mania.

Hygiene If the patient is unkempt, it might mean disorganised thinking or it might be a feature of a chronic disorder. Observe nails, hair and teeth.

Behaviour
Imagine you are watching a silent movie of the patient. Describe what you see.

Eye contact This is a non-specific indicator: poor eye contact can indicate something is wrong. It means you have to look for the problem. Just like a high temperature is non-specific, it means you have to try to find the cause. Be conscious of cultural issues.

Posture Slumped might indicate depression. Standing could mean the patient is anxious or irritable.

Movements Restlessness could mean the patient is anxious, irritated, scared or angry. Slow movements might indicate psychomotor retardation as occurs in depression. Extrapyramidal side-effects (EPSEs) are often the result of antipsychotics: look for Parkinsonism (pill rolling tremor of the hands), tardive dyskinesia (involuntary movements of the mouth), dystonia (often a spasm of the neck muscles) and akathisia (restless feet).

Speech

This aspect describes the mechanics of producing a voice, not what is said.

Rate A fast speech pattern might indicate mania or anxiety. Manic speech is pressured, i.e. uninterruptible. Slow speech could indicate depression.

Prosody This is the musicality of speech. Loss of prosody may indicate depression, chronic schizophrenia or drug side-effect.

Affect

Affect is a way of describing how you think the patient is feeling right now, in the room in front of you.

Quality This describes the type of emotion. Is the patient happy, sad, elevated, frustrated, angry, perplexed or something else?

Intensity A blunted affect feels like there is a pane of glass between you and the patient. This is a classical sign of chronic schizophrenia.

Range This describes how many emotions the patient has in the interview. We all go through a range of emotions in an hour, even if they are minor variations of emotions. The range can become restricted (i.e. only one or two emotions) in schizophrenia and depression.

Mobility This is how quickly the emotions accelerate. When labile, the affect can change from sad to buoyant in a matter of minutes—a characteristic of mania.

Reactivity Does the affect change according to what you say? If not then the affect is unreactive, which can indicate schizophrenia or depression.

Congruence When the affect doesn't fit the thought then it is said to be incongruent. For example, laughing when talking of the loss of a cherished parent. This can occur in mania and schizophrenia.

Thought

Stream This is how quickly the thoughts come out. Stream may be increased in mania, slowed in depression.

Form This is a description of how the thoughts are joined up. In simple terms, each sentence is a thought. Do the sentences (thoughts) flow logically from one to the next? If there is a problem then there may be a formal thought disorder (FTD). There are many types of FTD.

- **Tangentiality** is when the point is gradually lost as the patient speaks. For example, the patient is asked how they came to hospital: 'Well I was brought in by ambulance. Probably had a big engine, V8 with 5.6 litre capacity. The steering wasn't great. My old car had...' and they do not return to the point.
- **Derailment** is a more severe form of tangentiality. To the same question they might respond: 'An ambulance took me in. My house has blue walls. Dr Smith comes to the ward. Why does the TV have no speakers?' Both derailment and tangentiality are grouped under the heading of 'loosening of associations' (i.e. the associations between sentences) and are characteristic of acute psychosis.
- **Flight of ideas** is another FTD and characteristic of mania. Here each sentence is linked to the next one but the point rapidly shifts each time. For example: 'I came in by ambulance. They drove really fast. My dad drives so slowly. My dad drives as fast as a tortoise. There's a zoo around the corner with loads of reptiles.'
- **Circumstantiality** (or over-inclusiveness) is often a sign of anxiety or other disorder. It means providing way too much irrelevant detail in response to a question but eventually returning to the point.
- **Perseveration** is when the patient keeps returning to the same theme. For example, no matter what is asked of Doris, she steers the conversation back to her doll collection. It is characteristic of dementia.

Content This covers two areas: themes and pathology. Themes are basically the essence of what the patient is saying, for example, stress, pain, guilt, revenge, sadness, etc.

Pathology includes delusions, ideas of reference, passivity, obsessions or overvalued ideas.

Perception
Perception covers hallucinations, which can occur in any of the five senses.

Cognition
Cognition means 'thinking processes'. There are many tests of cognition. The most important things to comment on here are conscious state (alert or clouded) and orientation to date and place. Impaired cognition can be a feature of many psychiatric disorders. The type of impairment points to the type of the disorder. For example, frontal lobe deficits can occur in chronic schizophrenia; dementia tends to involve memory; delirium affects conscious state and orientation.

Insight
Does the patient know what is wrong and how it affects them?

Judgment
How capable is the patient of making decisions?

Rapport
Describe the relationship between you and the patient.

4

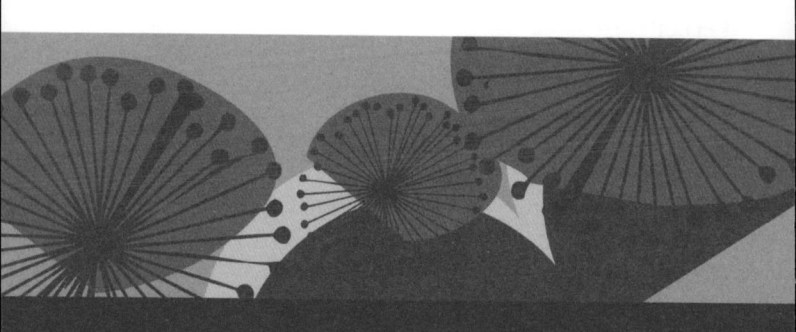

Making a diagnosis: proposing a formulation

CHAPTER 4 Making a diagnosis: proposing a formulation

For internal medicine, pathology mostly equates to diagnosis. For example, pneumococcal infection in the lungs = pneumonia; necrosed myocardium = myocardial infarction. But in psychiatry there are very few pathological entities that directly equate to a diagnosis. In psychiatry the diagnosis is made when there is a syndrome of symptoms and signs. That is, the diagnosis is made on history (symptoms) and mental state examination (signs).

The *Diagnostic and Statistical Manual of Mental Disorders* (see Chapter 1) has a list of the requisite symptoms and signs for each diagnosis.

THE INTERVIEW

Your job is to interview the patient and determine how their symptoms and signs fit together to make a diagnosis (or diagnoses). When taking the history you ask screening questions and if the screen is positive (e.g. 'Yes, I do feel sad a lot of the time') then you further explore that area to elicit more of the symptoms (in the above example, for depression). You then look for the signs (psychomotor retardation, monotone speech, etc.). By the end of the interview you come away with a list of symptoms and signs that may fit into a diagnostic category.

That all sounds fairly straightforward. However, complexity arises because while two patients may have the same diagnosis (say, depression), they may have very different symptoms and signs. Also, the myriad factors explaining their diagnosis can be very different. That's where the formulation comes in.

THE FORMULATION

In order to explain the complexities, nuances and contributions to a patient's presentation we make a formulation. A formulation is a statement (often several paragraphs long) that *hypothesises* an explanation as to why *this particular person*, presents in *this particular way* at *this particular time*.

For example, Jed, a 29 year old, is diagnosed as having major depression according to the DSM-IV. A brief formulation might look something like this:

Case study

Jed's early childhood was one of deprivation and loss. Parental conflict meant little time was spent caring for him and, consequently, he retreated to solitary activities. His treasured and only brother left home early, when Jed was only eight years old, leaving him to fend for himself. From the age of about ten he witnessed his mother's frequent episodes of depression. From his mother, Jed inherited a genetic risk for an affective disorder. His father abused alcohol, returning home intoxicated and sullen. At times his father would not return for days and his mother would be frantic. Likely, Jed internalised a view of the world as a harsh and lonely place imbued with a sense that at any time he may lose those close to him. Perhaps this may explain why Jed developed a fear that loved ones would leave. Jed's current reliance on alcohol can be thought of as modelling his father's behaviour. His relapse signature of depression is similar to his mother's, in that he stays in bed with the curtains drawn, relying on his wife for meals. His coping strategies are to seek reassurance and when it is not forthcoming he feels overwhelmed and unable to cope.

Recently Jed was diagnosed with hypertension. He was prescribed a beta-blocker and this coincided with his decline in mood; depression is a known potential side-effect of this medication. With the current economic downturn, there have been many retrenchments from Jed's accounting firm. It is clear that Jed is fearful that this may also be his fate. This occurs within the context of young man aiming to forge a career and with dreams of starting a family.

Fortunately for Jed he has a very supportive family and local church group. He is physically well and has fairly good insight into his condition. He has been adherent to management suggestions and is keen to engage in psychotherapy and take medication.

The formulation takes *facts*—such as Jed's beta-blocker use or his emotionally deprived childhood—and uses them to *explain* his current presentation. Because we can never really know if our explanation is correct, the formulation is always a hypothesis. It may change when you obtain more information.

WRITING A FORMULATION

How do you write a formulation? Use the table below to help you. Each dot point is a prompt to think about that factor for the patient. Is that factor present? If yes, circle it and write in the specifics. For example, for Jed you would circle 'Genetic' and write next to it 'family history of affective disorder—mother diagnosed with depression'; circle 'Modelling' and write next to it 'Jed witnessed father abusing alcohol as a means of dealing with stress'; and so on. Not all the dot points need be circled, only the relevant ones. The arrows indicate that the dot points from one box may also be relevant for another. Predisposing factors may also act to perpetuate.

Try to fill in the boxes one column at a time. Once you have entered as many factors as you can, start writing an explanation one row at a time—that is, going from predisposing (factors far back in time) to precipitating (current factors) then perpetuating (ongoing factors). How do the factors explain the presentation? End with the positives protectives. Remember this is just a theory.

What's the point of a formulation? It can help patients understand themselves and help you treat them because you understand the interaction of factors giving rise to their presentation. These factors can then be addressed in your treatment plan.

TABLE 4.1 Prompts for writing a formulation

	Biological	Psychological	Social
Predisposing	• Genetic • Birth trauma • Brain injury • Illness—psychiatric, physical • Medication • Drugs/alcohol • Pain	• Personality • Modelling • Defences (unconscious) • Coping strategies (conscious) • Self-esteem • Body image • Cognition	• Socioeconomic status • Trauma
Precipitating	• Medication • Trauma • Drugs/alcohol • Acute illness • Pain	• Stage of life • Loss/grief • Treatment • Stressors	• Work • Finances • Connections • Relationships
Perpetuating	↓	↓	↓
Protective	• Physical health	• Engagement • Insight • Adherence • Coping strategies • Intelligence	↓

5

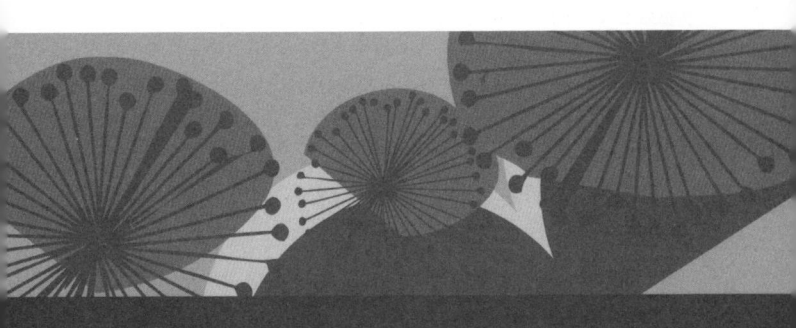

Risk assessment

In psychiatry, risk mostly refers to the potential for a patient to physically harm themselves or others. There are other types of risks: self-neglect, financial peril, exploitation by others, risk to reputation and absconding. In this chapter, we'll deal with assessing the risk of suicide.

PURPOSE OF THE RISK ASSESSMENT

There are very few absolutes in psychiatry; however, one of them is that every patient requires a risk assessment.

Just in case you didn't read that sentence:

Every patient requires a risk assessment.

For some patients the risk assessment may need to be very comprehensive, for others briefer, depending on context and presentation. But every patient requires a risk assessment.

At the end of a risk assessment you will *not* have a number or a percentage chance of that person coming to harm. Rather, a completed risk assessment paints a picture of the various aspects of the patient's situation and their disorder that colour the risk. A well-performed risk assessment has further important purposes: it provides an opportunity to explore helpful options; it can be a relief for the patient to unburden him or herself; and medico-legally, a thorough, written risk assessment is important documentation.

The risk assessment is taken as part of the history, but you need to be careful about when—it is confronting asking about ending one's life. You need to have established a rapport to get honest answers, so don't jump in too soon. Remember to listen first and be conscious of what may make the patient reluctant to talk (such as embarrassment, fear of consequences, being inarticulate about emotions, time pressure, paranoid delusions, thought disorder). Be non-judgmental and truthful about the limits of confidentiality. If a patient tells you something that puts them or others at risk, confidentiality does not necessarily apply.

MAKING THE RISK ASSESSMENT

A structured risk assessment involves the acronym **CHAIR**: **C**urrent statement, past **H**istory, **A**ttempt, **I**llnesses, **R**isk factors.

Current statement

What is the patient saying about their current wish to live or die?

Engage the patient in escalating questions:

'Do you feel that life is not worth living?'
'Would you rather be dead?'
'Do you think about killing yourself?' (This is suicidal ideation.)
'Do you plan on killing yourself? ... How?' (These are suicide plans.)

Roughly speaking, a low risk level statement involves thinking about suicide (but no plans or intention), a moderate statement is suicidal plans that are vague, unrealistic or unclear, and a high risk statement involves realistic plans with the intention to complete the suicide attempt.

Past history
The best predictor of future behaviour is past behaviour. The past history of suicide attempts, potential lethality and the consequences shape the current risk.

Attempt
How potentially lethal was the attempt? Did the patient expect to die? How lethal was the plan?

Did they carry through with the plan? Did they make efforts not to be stopped?

Illnesses
Think of psychiatric and medical illnesses.

Particularly high risks are depression, psychosis (especially if it involves command hallucinations to self-harm), drug and alcohol abuse and, in the hospital setting, delirium.

Medical illnesses are particularly risky if they involve chronic pain, are terminal or disfiguring or involve high care demands (e.g. dialysis).

Risk factors
Common high-risk factors include living in isolated or rural settings, divorce or separation, unemployment, a family history of suicide, and being male.

RISK MANAGEMENT
So, what do we do now that we've done a risk assessment? We manage the risk.

Management of risk is all about good **STAFF: S**afety, **T**reatment, **A**ttenuation of stressors, **F**ollow-up and **F**raternity.

Safety

Does the patient require containment in hospital? Sometimes involuntary admission (i.e. against their will) is necessary. Most places in the world have a mental health act of some sort—these are a set of laws that allow clinicians to treat patients with a mental illness who are a risk to themselves or others, even if the patient is not (or is not capable of) consenting.

If a decision is made to manage the patient in the community then it is important to garner as much support as possible. Carers should be involved. They can help with emotional support as well as medication adherence, appointments, contacting professionals, etc. A crisis team may be suitable to monitor and treat the patient. Other professionals involved should be contacted and following an agreed course of action so that care is consistent and each healthcare provider (e.g. GP, psychiatrist, psychologist, mental health nurse) knows their role. The plan in the community should be explicit about how often the patient is to be reviewed and by whom, and what circumstances merit what action.

Treatment

This doesn't mean medication alone. It means a bio-psycho-social approach. In the case of depression, treatment in the community might mean medication, psycho-education, counselling, vocational advice/rehabilitation, lifestyle advice, and enlisting the alliance of family, for example.

Attenuation of stressors

What is the meaning behind the suicidal feeling? Suicidal patients often feel that they have no other option, when in reality they aren't able to clearly see other solutions to their problems. They develop 'tunnel vision' so that suicide or self-harm seems to be the only solution. The key here is to open up other options.

Also, often a suicide attempt is a means of communicating distress. The key then is to listen to the patient as well as to encourage other ways of communicating distress.

The stressor itself may be a problem in a relationship, at work or at school, legal issues, problem with finances, sexuality concerns or physical illness. All these areas are amenable to some form of help. Be broad in thinking about what may lessen the stress.

Follow-up
Follow-up is imperative. A health professional must follow up the patient with a clear plan and goals.

Fraternity
Dealing with risk is stressful. It's important to have peers or seniors to talk to and share the load. As a student you should *never* be in a situation where you alone assess risk. An experienced clinician should *always* be taking the lead.

6

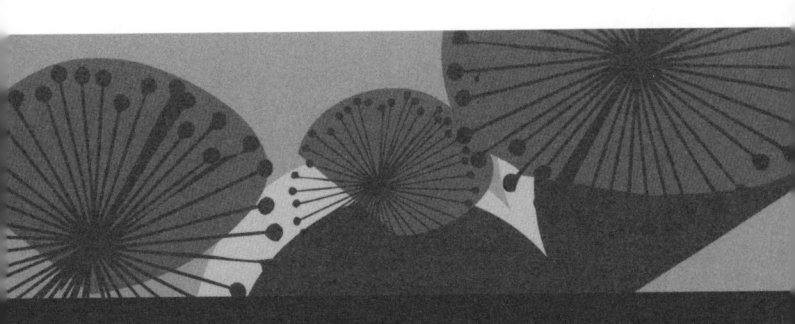

Mood disorders

There are two moods that are of major interest to psychiatry: depression and mania. When depression occurs alone it is called a **depressive disorder**, but if the person has experienced an episode of mania (now or in the past), it is called **bipolar disorder** (the old name was manic–depressive disorder). Depression is common—one in five people experience it at some stage in their life—while bipolar disorder is rare (lifetime prevalence about 1 per cent).

Depression is by far the commonest psychiatric disorder that doctors treat, and no matter what area of medicine you choose, it will be a part of your working life (so get good at it!).

DEPRESSION

Everyone gets sad and depressed from time to time so, as with all psychiatry, we have to set cut-off points to distinguish normal sadness from clinical or major depression. The rule of thumb from the American Psychiatric Association *Diagnostic and Statistical Manual of Mental Disorders* (DSM-IV) is five or more symptoms for at least two weeks, with a significant impairment in social or occupational functioning. In reality, most people you see will have had depression for far longer than just two weeks.

The nine key symptoms are:

1. Lowered mood
2. Lack of enjoyment in usual activities (called anhedonia)
3. Change in eating pattern
4. Change in sleep pattern

5. Fatigue
6. Feeling worthless or guilty
7. Poor concentration
8. Feeling agitated or slowed up
9. Recurrent thoughts of death or suicide.

Key features to look for on mental state examination are a depressed affect that lacks reactivity. The person may be tearful; they may have psychomotor retardation and monotone speech. There may be suicidal ideas or plans.

The causes of depression are many and varied, and include biological factors (e.g. medical illnesses, drugs, hereditary factors), psychological factors (e.g. difficult childhood, abuse, multiple losses) and social factors (e.g. isolation, relationship problems, stress).

Most people (about 80 per cent) recover from a depressive episode, usually after about six months of treatment. Unfortunately, at least half will have another episode, and many have recurrent episodes throughout their life.

There is also a subtype of depression called **dysthymia,** which is a chronic mild depression lasting at least two years, but not fulfilling the criteria for major depression.

It is very important to think of comorbidity with depression. Think: anxiety disorders, drug and alcohol disorders, somatisation and pain disorders. Most people with depression have one of these factors interacting with their depression in some way.

The most feared outcome of depression is suicide. While we know that depression is common in those who complete suicide, the precise risk of suicide in a depressed person is difficult to determine. In severe depression the risk is probably around 10 per cent (i.e. very high).

BIPOLAR DISORDER

In bipolar disorder the person has recurrent episodes of depression and mania.

A manic episode is a distinct period of elevated mood lasting at least a week causing marked impairment in functioning. Sometimes the mood is more irritable than elevated, and because their mood is labile (i.e. it fluctuates) mania can occasionally be mistaken for depression. The associated symptoms include grandiosity, decreased sleep, increased talkativeness, distractibility, agitation and involvement in high-risk activities for pleasure. Mania is dramatic and overwhelming when you first see it—the sufferers are larger than life, taking all sorts of risks and raising all sorts of feelings (from distress to humour) in others. When severe, they are delusional, such that it is hard to distinguish mania from acute schizophrenia.

Mania usually occurs as part of bipolar disorder, but can occur secondary to medical illnesses, typically disorders that damage the brain, such as dementia and advanced HIV.

TREATMENT
Depression

Think of depression treatment in five phases:

1. Confirm the diagnosis: investigate underlying causes and explore comorbidity.
2. Explain the diagnosis and begin the continuing process of education.
3. Basic psychological first aid: discuss the importance of stress management, exercise, relaxation, reducing substance use (alcohol, drugs and caffeine), relationships, work, and provide support.

4. Psychotherapy—the main psychotherapy for depression is cognitive behaviour therapy. It works in about 70 per cent of depressive episodes, takes about one hour per week for three months and seems to be associated with fewer relapses than medications.
5. Medications—there are many antidepressant drugs available. They are all similar in effectiveness, onset of action and tolerability. They work in about 65 per cent of episodes. If one trial doesn't work, we switch to another class, usually after being sure of compliance for at least four weeks.

The choice of treatment is fairly simple: in mild depression (i.e. just makes the criteria, no suicidal ideas) we recommend phases 1 to 3. In moderate depression (six or seven symptoms, suicide risk is low) phases 1 to 3 plus psychotherapy and/or medications (usually based on the patient's choice). In severe depression treatment should encompass all five phases, and consideration given to hospitalising the patient if the suicide risk is significant (a psychiatric referral should be made).

Bipolar disorder

Bipolar disorder treatment needs to be thought of in three phases:

1. Treatment of depressive episodes
2. Treatment of manic episodes
3. Prevention of further episodes.

Treatment of depressive episodes

The treatment of a depressive episode is essentially the same as for depression without bipolar disorder as described above, except that we usually do not prescribe antidepressants alone, as they can trigger manic episodes. So if medications are needed, we start with a mood stabiliser, and if that isn't enough, add an antidepressant later.

Treatment of manic episodes

Mania rarely settles without medications and, in fact, usually gets worse.

There are two classes of drugs to consider: antipsychotics and mood stabilisers. Sometimes a combination is used. Benzodiazepines (e.g. diazepam) are often added, especially to help with sleep and to slow motor symptoms.

Prevention of further episodes

Mood stabilisers decrease the frequency of further episodes (they rarely stop them altogether). Historically, lithium was the first of these prescribed, and is effective, but requires close monitoring of levels, so is less favoured. Anti-epileptic medications are now favoured, with the most popular being sodium valproate and carbamazepine. Patients need to stay on these long term.

Reference

American Psychiatric Association 1994, *Diagnostic and Statistical Manual of Mental Disorders*, 4th edn, American Psychiatric Association, Washington DC.

7

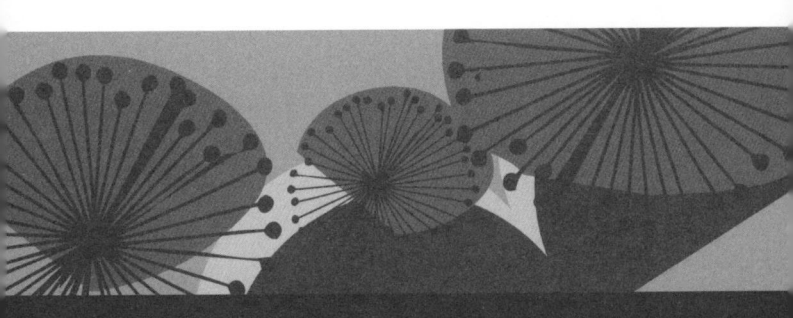

Schizophrenia

Schizophrenia is an important disorder for you to know as it can have a wide range of effects for the individual, the family and the community. Schizophrenia affects approximately 1 per cent of the population (this number is remarkably consistent across most cultures and geographies). It is equally common in males and females; however, it affects men and women at different stages of life.

The age of onset is usually in the late teens for males and mid to late twenties for females. There is also a second peak age for females, just after menopause. When schizophrenia onsets at this age it is called 'late onset' schizophrenia or **paraphrenia**.

DIAGNOSIS

Schizophrenia does not mean split personality. *Schizo* means break and *phrenia*, mind—literally, 'a break in the mind', but more correctly, in *reality testing*. When reality testing is impaired the patient is said to have a **psychosis**.

A psychosis is identified clinically when one (or more) of the following is present:

- Hallucinations
- Delusions
- Formal thought disorder
- Catatonia.

Psychosis can occur as part of a number of disorders (e.g. bipolar disorder, delirium, drug intoxication) but it is the hallmark feature of schizophrenia.

A **hallucination** is defined as a sensation in the absence of a stimulus, i.e. perceiving something that is not really there. In schizophrenia the hallucinations are most often auditory (in the form of voices). **Command hallucinations** are voices instructing the patient to perform an act. They can be dangerous, for example, instructing the patient to self-harm. Hallucinations in other senses, such as visual or olfactory hallucinations, do occur in schizophrenia, but can sometimes point to organic pathology as well, such as drug intoxication, brain tumours or epilepsy.

A **delusion** is defined as a belief (or thought) that is false, fixed and out of keeping with social, cultural and educational context. Delusions can be of different types. Paranoid or persecutory delusions refer to the belief that one is being targeted by an individual or group. While one may indeed be a target (rarely in clinical practice, though) it is the evidence on which the beliefs are based that is important. In persecutory delusions there is no real evidence. Grandiose delusions are those involving one's greatness. Morbid jealously is a delusion involving a partner's perceived infidelity. Any of these delusions can occur in schizophrenia but persecutory delusions are the most common.

Catatonia is an uncommon movement disorder that can occur in patients with a psychosis (schizophrenia in particular). The patient either presents with a loss of spontaneous movement or demonstrates too much movement. In the former, patients can hold a rigid posture for hours, oblivious to external stimulation; in the latter, patients are extremely overactive. Both types of catatonia are very serious conditions as they can be fatal if untreated.

Clinically, when a young person first presents with a psychosis, a diagnosis of **first episode psychosis** is given

(FEP). That's because the psychosis might be due to a substance intoxication/withdrawal, evolve into an affective disorder (bipolar disorder, for example), or be the beginnings of schizophrenia. In the case of schizophrenia, there is often a history of a year or so of a *prodrome*. In that period, according to others, the patient will often have undergone a change in personality. The patient is likely to have become socially isolated, hold odd ideas, used (more) illicit drugs, had distressing mood symptoms and/or muddled thinking.

The diagnosis of schizophrenia is only made when the symptoms have been present for six months or more and there is no other explanation for their cause. There are *positive* and *negative* symptoms of schizophrenia. Positive symptoms are the same as psychotic symptoms. They tend to be most prominent at the onset of the disorder or during acute exacerbations. Negative symptoms are losses. They evolve after many years of schizophrenia, especially if not optimally treated. Social withdrawal, blunted affect, poverty of speech, anhedonia and amotivation are typical negative symptoms. Cognitive symptoms of schizophrenia can be prominent and tend to co-occur with the negative symptoms. The cognitive symptoms typically involve the frontal lobe, so tasks such as planning, organisation, verbal fluency and abstracting can be impaired.

Untreated, psychotic episodes of schizophrenia can last months or years. Some of the potential consequences of untreated psychosis include: self-neglect; exploitation by others; risk to self or others; making decisions based on psychotic beliefs (e.g. moving towns under the pain of paranoid beliefs); and damage to relationships, education and careers. Thus it is imperative that treatment be offered as soon as possible.

Treatment can be difficult as patients with a psychosis may not believe they are unwell. Moreover, they may believe that healthcare workers or even family are part of the conspiracy to hurt them. That's one reason why some patients you see on the ward or in the community may be involuntary patients.

MANAGEMENT

Management of a patient with schizophrenia really needs to cover the broad gamut of bio-psycho-social management. That is, medications are necessary but insufficient by themselves. Patients require a multidisciplinary approach. Family work, vocational and/or educational rehabilitation, psychological support and psycho-education are important parts of the management. Having a relapse prevention plan is vital. Case management can provide a range of services such as advocacy, service brokerage, risk review and many others. Social engagement is important and this can be via services such as social skills training, support groups and/or non-disability-specific groups.

MEDICATION

The medications used are called anti-psychotics (the old name was major tranquillisers). There are a number of different types, each with different side-effect profiles; they are covered in Chapter 12. The sooner treatment is started, the shorter the duration of the psychosis, and the better the prognosis. However, if medications are started without adequate explanation and family/carer support, one risks non-compliance. The medications can be given in various forms: oral tablets or injectable 'depot' style for patients in whom adherence is problematic (depots can last for up to a month).

8

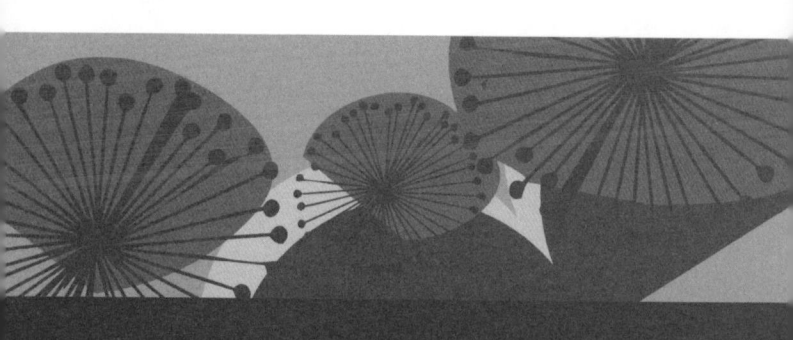

Anxiety disorders

Anxiety is an emotion we are all familiar with, and the anxiety disorders are probably the most common psychiatric disorders.

OVERVIEW
Before we go anywhere with this topic, try to put into words how *you* would define anxiety. Stop for a minute and have a think before reading on (feeling a bit anxious?).

Despite being experienced by us all, anxiety is hard to define. Anxiety is similar to fear and apprehension but usually occurs in response to an *anticipated* problem or hazard. The components of anxiety can be divided into:

- Psychological (feelings)—feeling frightened, irritable and distractible
- Somatic (physical)—many and varied, but typically including palpitations, racing pulse, hyperventilation, dizziness, nausea and diarrhoea
- Cognitive (thoughts)—a range of fearful thoughts, especially fear of losing control or going mad.

When anxiety is severe and gets to the stage of being called a *disorder* it tends to present in fairly typical syndromes (patterns). These are described below.

Panic disorder
Panic disorder is characterised by recurrent panic attacks often followed by months of persistent concern about more attacks. Panic attacks are sudden, unexpected attacks of

multiple anxiety symptoms that are not necessarily linked to any cue. Sufferers can think they are dying, so they may call an ambulance and be rushed to hospital. Agoraphobia often develops, which is the fear of being in places or situations from which escape may be difficult (e.g. crowds or shopping centres). This leads to avoidance of many types of activities.

Phobias

Phobias are an extreme form of fear related to a specific object or situation. The key here is that the fear is extreme and unreasonable. For example, most of us are afraid of spiders, but the fear would only be a phobia if the mere mention sent you into a panic and it disrupted your life in some way (if you threw down this book at the mention of a spider then you are in the ball park!). One of the commonest phobias is social phobia, which is so common it gets its own name (**social anxiety disorder**). Social phobia is the fear of any situation where public scrutiny may be possible, usually with the fear of having a panic attack, or behaving in a way that is embarrassing or humiliating.

Obsessive compulsive disorder

In obsessive compulsive disorder (OCD), specific cognitive and behavioural symptoms accompany the feelings of anxiety. These include obsessional thoughts (recurrent thoughts, impulses or images that are experienced as intrusive and inappropriate and that cause marked anxiety), and compulsions (repetitive behaviours or mental acts that the person feels driven to perform in response to an obsession and in order to reduce anxiety).

OCD is usually a chronic illness, with a waxing and waning course. The most frequent presenting obsessions are those related to contamination and doubt (e.g. 'Did I turn off the stove?'). Frequent compulsions include the need to wash, check and count. The diagnosis of OCD should be made when the symptoms are severe, persistent and distressing.

Post-traumatic stress disorder

As the name suggests, post-traumatic stress disorder (PTSD) occurs following a trauma. Symptoms include re-experiencing the trauma (e.g. recurrent dreams of the event or flashbacks), persistent avoidance of reminders of the trauma, and persistent symptoms of increased arousal (hypervigilence, irritability, exaggerated startle response). A diagnosis of PTSD is made if the symptoms are present for at least one month and cause significant distress or impairment in functioning.

Generalised anxiety disorder

Generalised anxiety disorder (GAD) is excessive anxiety and worry, occurring most days for more than six months. It essentially refers to excessive anxiety in a range of situations that does not fit into any of the above syndromes.

NORMAL VERSUS PATHOLOGICAL ANXIETY

The first and biggest problem you will face when confronted with a patient with anxiety is determining whether the anxiety is normal or not. As a rule of thumb, if the patient says it is severe and interrupting their life and they want treatment, then we call it a disorder (or 'pathological' anxiety). This point often irritates newcomers to psychiatry. Just remember that the rest of medicine isn't really that much more exact. You will hear similar debates in nearly all areas of illness, from cancer to hypertension.

PRIMARY VERSUS SECONDARY ANXIETY

Once you've established that a patient has an anxiety disorder, you must ask yourself whether it is primary or secondary. Secondary anxiety means it is caused by something else, either another medical condition or a drug. The common medical conditions are disorders of the thyroid and parathyroid, seizure disorders and cardiac conditions. The common drugs are amphetamines, cocaine, caffeine, salbutamol and steroids.

It is also true that anxiety can result from other psychiatric conditions, especially depression. If the anxiety only occurs in the context of the other psychiatric condition, we tend not to diagnose the anxiety disorder separately, but if it occurs both with and without the other disorder we will call it a comorbid condition.

TREATMENT

There is a basic formula for the treatment of all anxiety disorders:

1. Rule out secondary causes of anxiety—perform physical examination and laboratory tests.
2. Provide information—this is often called psycho-education; explain what is going on! (This in itself is arguably the best thing you can do!)
3. Basic psychological first aid—give diet, exercise, relaxation skills, relationship and lifestyle (work) advice where appropriate. Also recommend decreased caffeine intake.
4. Psychological therapy—the commonest is cognitive behaviour therapy, but there are others. The specific techniques vary for the different anxiety disorders.

5. Medications—All antidepressants are also anti-anxiety drugs (but they can take many weeks to work). Benzodiazepines (e.g. diazepam) work within half an hour but issues with dependence limit their long-term use to (ideally) less than two weeks.

For mild anxiety disorders, provide options 1 to 3. For moderate disorders, provide options 1 to 3 plus a choice of options 4 or 5 (patient preference, some choose both), and for severe disorders recommend all five options.

9

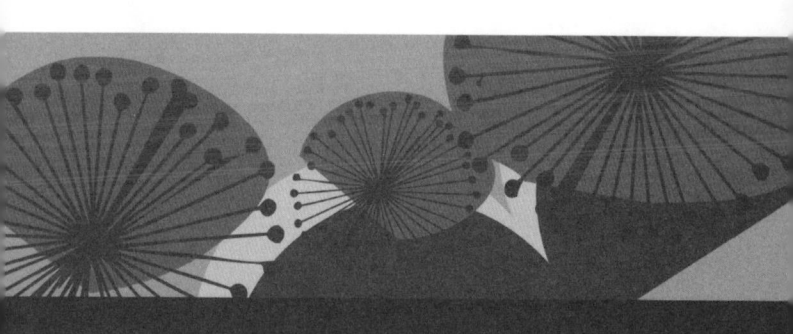

Drug and alcohol disorders

Drugs and alcohol (D & A) have an impact on nearly all areas of medicine. Psychiatry is just one of the specialties that take an interest in these disorders. In recent decades D & A has become a specialty area in its own right.

KEY ASPECTS

From a psychiatric perspective, there are three key aspects to this topic. Firstly, drugs and alcohol can cause their own problems: intoxication, withdrawal, abuse and dependence. Secondly, drugs and alcohol can cause other psychiatric problems (e.g. amphetamines can cause a psychosis). Finally, you need to know a little about the drugs themselves.

Intoxication

This is the acute effects of taking the drug. Each drug has a different intoxication profile. Most drugs cause some sort of intoxication. Alcohol intoxication, for example, has typical signs of slurred speech, poor coordination, unsteady gait, impaired attention and sedation. Some students have been observed to experience these effects themselves on occasion.

Withdrawal

This is the syndrome that results from stopping a drug after prolonged use. It can even occur after simply reducing the dose. Not all drugs cause a withdrawal syndrome. Like intoxication, the withdrawal syndrome is specific to the drug. For example, alcohol withdrawal comes on after about 6 to 24 hours, and causes autonomic hyperactivity, tremor, insomnia, agitation, hallucinations and sometimes even seizures.

Abuse

Abuse refers to a maladaptive pattern of drug use, such that the person's functioning deteriorates as a consequence of the drug use, or they use it in a hazardous way (e.g. while driving), or they suffer recurrent legal problems. Hence, it refers to the lifestyle that can go along with drug use.

Dependence

Dependence refers to the severe end of the drug use spectrum. There is a mix of tolerance (needing more drug to get the same effect), withdrawal, using more of the drug than initially intended, persistent and unsuccessful efforts to cut back usage, and persistent use despite knowing it is doing harm.

Note that the term **addiction** is *not* a disorder in this classification. Addiction has a different meaning to different people, and is used broadly in society. In medicine, addiction is roughly equivalent to dependence.

THE DRUGS

Each of these drugs has textbooks written about them. The goal here is to know the key points of relevance to psychiatry.

Alcohol

In most countries where you will work, alcohol will be legal (under certain conditions). The intoxication and withdrawal syndromes have already been mentioned. Alcohol dependence is the most common dependence treated in medicine. In psychiatry, we regularly treat withdrawal syndromes, and we often treat aspects of abuse and dependence. We also get involved in the psychiatric comorbidity. Anxiety disorders predispose to alcohol abuse, as sufferers may self-medicate with alcohol to reduce anxiety. Depression is also common in people who have alcohol dependence.

Cannabis

The effects vary, but include a sense of relaxation, reduced concentration, distorted perceptions of time, space and distance, drowsiness, poor coordination and increased appetite. There has been an ongoing debate about the links between cannabis use and schizophrenia. The current belief is that it exacerbates schizophrenia by causing relapses and can precipitate schizophrenia in people who are predisposed.

Amphetamines

Amphetamines are a group of related synthetic stimulant drugs. There are legal forms (dexamphetamine, methylphenidate) used for medical purposes (narcolepsy and attention deficit disorder) and illegal forms (mostly methamphetamine). A stronger form of methamphetamine called 'ice' is also popular in some groups of society. Amphetamines stimulate the sympathetic nervous system, causing increased heart rate and blood pressure and adrenaline release. In small doses they increase alertness and make the user feel refreshed, energetic, more talkative and excited. In high doses they cause extreme anxiety, agitation, confusion and irritability often leading to aggression. Intoxication is a common emergency department presentation. Dependence is also common. Typical psychiatric problems include psychosis with intoxication, depression with continued use, and a range of other health and social problems.

Opioids

The commonest illicit opioid is heroin, but in recent years this has been overtaken by abuse of the prescribed opioids. Opioids are central nervous system depressants. They slow breathing and decrease blood pressure and body temperature. Unconsciousness with high doses is common. Nausea and vomiting is common. The beneficial effect is a rush of extremely pleasurable feelings.

There are a number of problems for health care. Firstly, overdose—people often take too much, fall into a coma and can die. Secondly, dependence—tolerance builds quickly, and the withdrawal syndrome is strong, hence there is a high rate of dependence compared to other drugs. Withdrawal comes on quickly and includes cravings, diarrhoea, vomiting, sweating, various pains and depression. The social consequences can be dramatic in the effort to obtain more drugs. There are also myriad physical consequences related to unhealthy injection technique and the consequences of the lifestyle. Finally, there is the challenge of sensible prescribing of opioids versus prescribing that contributes to dependence.

Cocaine

Cocaine is a stimulant that can be snorted or injected. There is also a form that can be smoked, called 'crack'. It causes feelings of euphoria and confidence. Physical effects include a rapid heart rate, increased body temperature, increased energy and the urge to have sex. Overdose is a common problem. While tolerance is not a major problem, withdrawal can last for months. Dependence is common. Psychotic symptoms can occur when intoxicated, and mood and anxiety symptoms are common during withdrawal.

Ecstasy

Methylenedioxymethamphetamine (MDMA) is both a stimulant and a hallucinogen. It is a tablet taken orally. It causes feeling of confidence, happiness and benevolence. It can increase blood pressure and heart rate, and cause sweating and dehydration. The drug is mostly made in backyard laboratories, so the dose is unknown, and overdose is common and can be fatal. When used for extended periods, depression and panic attacks are common, and psychotic symptoms may develop.

Other drugs

There are many other drugs that will be the focus of your attention from time to time. Just be aware of them, and gradually build your knowledge. Don't forget the legal drugs (caffeine, nicotine and prescription drugs such as sedatives).

10

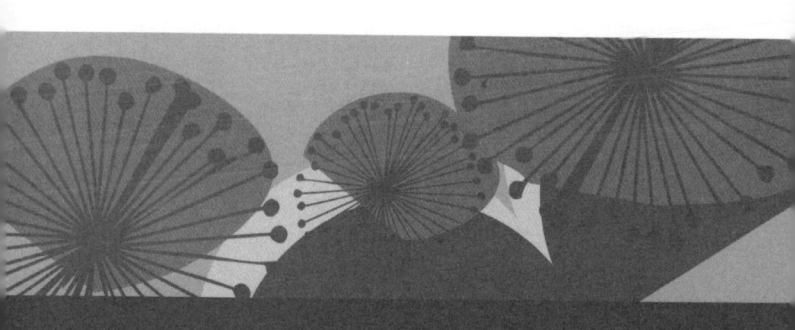

Personality disorders

Personality is an individual's unique pattern of thoughts, feelings, behaviours and styles of interacting in the world that endures over time (i.e. it doesn't change much or, if it does, it changes slowly).

Personality descriptions are important to psychiatrists because many patients present with difficulties arising from personality factors.

THE DEVELOPMENT OF PERSONALITY

The ancient Greeks believed that personality was determined by one's 'humours' or fluids. So they named them after each: melancholic (sad, via an excess of black bile); sanguine (cheerful, a surplus of blood); choleric (assertive, lots of yellow bile); and phlegmatic (stoic, loads of phlegm). While these words are descriptive, we know through modern science that the causes they are based on are unlikely!

Today we conceptualise personality as being made up of a number of different traits (pronounced *trays*). There are many different traits described (e.g. impulsivity, obsessionality, aggression, etc.). We each have a unique combination of different traits in varying amounts.

There are many theories about how personality traits develop. There are some genetic links, for example, it comes as no surprise that males (XY) tend to aggression more than females (XX). There are also many psychological theories about childhood experiences. Most people think that some traits are biological and some are learnt (nature and nurture). By and large, personality is largely established by the time of adulthood.

Sometimes personality traits are adaptive. For example, having obsessional traits is useful for work as a librarian or accountant. Dramatic traits are useful for performers. A personality disorder exists when the traits are significantly maladaptive. For example, being disproportionately dramatic so that friends and family are driven away, as can happen in histrionic personality disorder. Or expecting an unreasonably high level of orderliness, thus aggravating work colleagues and housemates, as can happen in obsessive compulsive personality disorder.

CLASSIFICATION OF PERSONALITY DISORDERS

DSM-IV divides personality disorders into three categories (or clusters): clusters A, B and C. Cluster A contains the personality disorders that are typified by oddness or eccentricity. Cluster A disorders are: schizoid, schizotypal and paranoid personality disorders. Cluster B personality disorders are dramatic, emotional or erratic. Patients with cluster B personality disorders often draw attention from mental health services because they can have a dramatic presentation with significant consequences for themselves and others (e.g. a suicide attempt). Cluster B disorders are: borderline, antisocial, narcissistic and histrionic personality disorders. Cluster C personality disorders have anxiety or fear as a core feature. Cluster C disorders are: dependant, avoidant and obsessive compulsive personality disorders.

BORDERLINE PERSONALITY DISORDER

Borderline personality disorder (BPD) is important to know about because it is often associated with marked distress and patients often have self-harm and/or suicide attempts.

CHAPTER 10 Personality disorders

They may have many psychiatric and medical comorbidities and it is one of the most common personality disorders seen in public psychiatry. DSM-IV covers nine potential traits for BPD:

1. Relationship instability—others are seen as either all good or all bad. New relationships are very intense
2. Abandonment fears—an intense fear of being left by friends, family, intimates and/or therapists
3. Impulsivity—such as buying sprees, drug use, imprudent relationships
4. Suicidal behaviour or self-harm—there is a history of repeated self-harm or suicidal behaviour
5. Emptiness—a chronic sense of feeling unfulfilled
6. Mood instability—mood can change over days or hours, for example, from profoundly sad to cheerful
7. Anger—can be intense and out of proportion to the provocation
8. Identity disturbance—not knowing one's aims, drives, career direction, etc.
9. Dissociation—not being 'present' or aware of the surroundings. This is especially so during a stressful time and/or around periods of self-harm. This may escalate into a brief episode of psychosis.

You can remember the criteria with the mnemonic: RAISE MAID

Aetiology

The aetiology of BPD is multi-factorial. It is more common in women than in men (the converse of anti-social personality disorder). Childhood sexual abuse is common in the developmental history. Psychodynamic theories place emphasis on the early home environment. For example, perceived parental neglect could engender a hypervigilance to abandonment, which might extend into adulthood.

TREATMENT

The treatment of personality disorders can be protracted and difficult. You can imagine that undoing decades-long patterns is not easy. Psychotherapies are the key in the long-term treatment of BPD. A psychotherapy specific for BPD is dialectical behaviour therapy (DBT). This effective, structured program includes teaching patients to tolerate distress and behaviour change through careful analysis of actions. DBT has a clear evidence base. In terms of medication, antidepressants can be used to treat low mood and impulsivity. Sodium valproate can be useful especially for rapid mood shifts. Antipsychotics have also been used to treat distress.

Other personality disorders are also treated by psychotherapy, albeit different styles. The challenge here is that the patient must be motivated to change, have sufficient insight, time and resources, and have the capacity for (often painful) self-reflection. You can imagine that while some fortunate people do, there are many people who do not have all or some of these.

Reference

American Psychiatric Association 1994, *Diagnostic and Statistical Manual of Mental Disorders*, 4th edn, American Psychiatric Association, Washington DC.

11

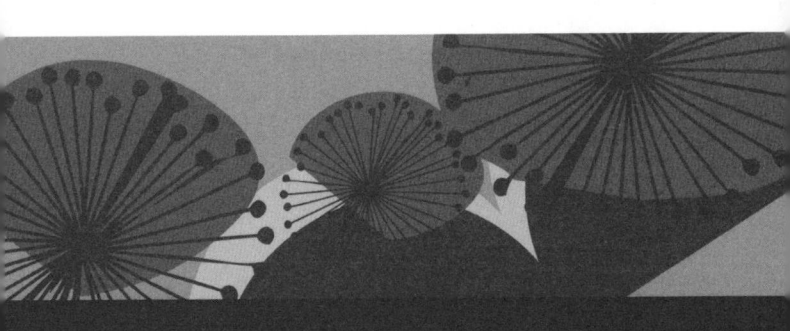

Consultation-liaison psychiatry

Consultation-liaison (C-L) psychiatry is a subspecialty of psychiatry in general hospital settings.

ROLE OF THE C-L PSYCHIATRIST

C-L psychiatrists have many roles. They manage the psychiatric disorders in sick patients (for example, if a patient with cancer also has schizophrenia); they manage the psychological consequences of medical illnesses (for example, depression in a patient with cancer, hallucinations after brain injury, post-traumatic stress disorder after a car crash); they help with the behavioural aspects of medical problems (such as a delirious patient who has become aggressive) and they help sort out ethical problems (Is the patient with cancer refusing treatment for well-considered personal reasons or because they are depressed and have a death wish?).

SPECIAL PROBLEMS IN C-L PSYCHIATRY

C-L psychiatrists see all sorts of psychiatric problems, and mostly apply the techniques and expertise from other areas of psychiatry into the hospital environment. There are two problems that are worth special mention because they both occur almost exclusively in the C-L setting.

Depression in the medically ill

Depression is common in the general population, and one of the most common times to get depressed is when you are sick. Illnesses that are chronic, are painful, potentially fatal or involve the brain are particularly likely to cause depression.

Depression in medically ill patients poses a number of challenges. Diagnosis is challenging—many of the symptoms of depression overlap with physical illness, especially poor sleep, low energy, poor concentration, weight change and thoughts about death. Hence, diagnosis is much more difficult. Often the doctor must delve far deeper into the symptoms to distinguish between depression and the underlying physical problem. A greater emphasis on examining the psychological symptoms of depression is helpful (for example, feeling worthless, guilty and a failure). Differentiating depression from normal grief can also be hard. Furthermore, many drugs used to treat the physical problem can cause depression, especially steroids and cancer drugs.

When depression is present, treatment can be challenging. Some antidepressants may interact with medical drugs, and psychotherapy is much harder if a patient is in hospital. Finally worth mentioning is the challenge of differentiating a death wish (suicidal thinking) with refusing life-saving treatment. This is complex, and not for the beginner to psychiatry, but to get you started the key questions are:

- Does the person understand what is happening?
- Is their cognitive function good enough to handle the decisions (are they competent)?
- Is the person really depressed?
- Are there other psychiatric disorders present?
- What was the person's view about treatment before getting sick, and before becoming mentally unwell?
- What do their loved ones say—is the patient's desire to stop treatment consistent with their past beliefs?

Somatoform disorders

The somatoform disorders are a fascinating group of problems in which the patient complains of physical symptoms that suggest major medical illnesses, yet have no associated serious, demonstrable organic basis for the symptoms *and* in which psychological factors seem to be playing a major role. Obviously, these disorders present to non-psychiatrists first—the patient believes they have a physical problem and, in fact, sometimes patients resent the psychiatrist being called in. Most doctors have seen patients with these disorders and most agree the management can be challenging. As a beginner, all you need to master are the key definitions.

Conversion disorder

These are medical symptoms caused by psychological factors. The symptoms are usually neurological, like losing the ability to move an arm. The cause is unconscious (the patient is *not* feigning), and usually the neurological signs don't make anatomical sense (e.g. complete loss of power in both legs, but with normal reflexes, tone and sensation). The patients often seem far less distressed by the symptom than would be expected—known as *la belle indifference*.

Hypochondriasis

This is a preoccupation with the fear of having a disease based on the misinterpretation of bodily symptoms that persists despite adequate reassurance. Of course we all have a little of this from time to time, especially while studying diseases (watch out, medical students!), so we don't call hypochondriasis a disorder until it has been causing significant problems for at least six months.

Somatisation disorder

This is the most prominent and severe of the somatoform disorders. It refers to a pattern of recurring physical complaints occurring over many years. The symptoms are not fully explained by medical illnesses, and they result in a range of often unnecessary investigations and treatments. Symptoms often include pain, pseudoneurological symptoms (conversion symptoms), sexual symptoms and gastrointestinal symptoms.

The main differential diagnosis for all these problems is some sort of organic pathology that has been missed. This is a real challenge clinically, because there are many medical problems that are hard to diagnose. The key in making the somatoform diagnosis is to look for the psychological cause. Remember, these are disorders in which psychological factors seem to be important. If you can't find a stress or a psychological cause, keep a very open mind.

The other differential diagnosis is that the patient is feigning their symptoms. There are two situations in which a patient feigns symptoms—factitious disorder (previously called Münchausen syndrome) and malingering.

These are not somatoform disorders. In factitious disorder the patient's reason is unclear; it appears to have no more purpose than to be in hospital or to be a patient, often called the desire to assume the sick role. In malingering, the purpose is to achieve some clear gain, such as money (financial compensation), time off work or something else.

Obviously this whole area is hard! Is the symptom organically based but elusive, is it an unconscious response to a psychological stress or is it being feigned—and if so, why? You need to be a clever physician, an astute psychiatrist and an amateur detective—not always an easy path to walk.

12

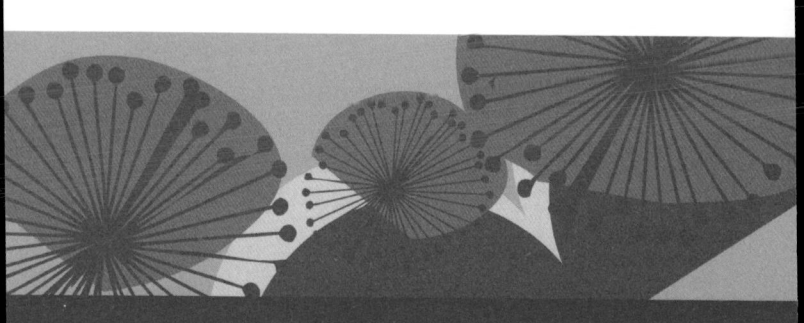

Medications

CHAPTER 12 Medications

Medications in psychiatry attract a lot of controversy. This isn't surprising because using medications to alter our emotions and thinking strikes at the core of who we are, and changing who we are is not as simple as using an antibiotic to kill a bacteria. Nevertheless, psychiatric medications have helped millions of people overcome severe problems and lead fulfilling lives. Our job is to help patients choose the right medication and use it in the right way.

TYPES OF MEDICATION

Medications in psychiatry are pretty straightforward. There are four main classes:

- Antidepressants
- Antipsychotics
- Anti-anxiety (also called anxiolytics)
- Mood stabilisers.

Even though each class consists of many medications, the medications within each class are *fairly* similar and *mostly* have similar efficacy and onset of action. The main differences are the side-effect profiles.

All have problems with efficacy and unwanted side effects, and some even cause dependence and withdrawal syndromes.

Before launching into an explanation of the four classes, there are a few things to note that apply to all the drugs:

- Non-adherence is a big problem in psychiatry, so always assess the patient's attitude to medications.

- Each class is used for multiple problems, so just because it is called an 'antidepressant' doesn't mean depression is its only indication (they are also used for anxiety, pain and other problems).
- All are slow to start working (except benzodiazepines), so patients need lots of information and reassurance to ensure they don't quit before the benefits begin.
- Drug interactions are common, so we start just one drug at a time and, where possible, start at a low dose and increase slowly.
- All have side effects and many cannot be used in pregnancy, so patients require lots of information about the risks and benefits.

ANTIDEPRESSANT MEDICATIONS

Major uses: depression (if moderate or severe), anxiety disorders, pain syndromes, insomnia and bulimia nervosa.

Common examples: citalopram, fluoxetine, fluvoxamine, paroxetine, sertraline (the SSRIs—selective serotonin re-uptake inhibitors), venlafaxine, mirtazepine, reboxetine.

Key things to know:
- They all take about two to six weeks to work.
- They are all equally effective (approximately 65 per cent response rate, compared to 35 per cent placebo response rate in depression).
- The choice of antidepressant is based on past response (the best predictor of the future is the past!) and side-effect profile.
- Ensure patients understand that:
  - Antidepressants are slow to work and the side effects come before the good effects (if we

don't warn patients of this they **will** stop the medications).
- They must take the drug every day.
- Once the symptoms improve the patient must stay on the medication for 6 to 12 months to prevent relapse (even longer if it's a recurrent episode).

ANTIPSYCHOTIC MEDICATIONS

Major uses: schizophrenia and related disorders, delirium, mania, and behavioural disturbances in the elderly. Sometimes also used for augmentation of antidepressants when the depression is refractory or has psychotic features.

Common examples: aripiprazole, clozapine, olanzepine, risperidone, ziprasidone (these are the newer drugs and are known as *atypicals*), chlorpromazine, haloperidol, thioridazine (these are the older drugs and are known as the *typical* antipsychotics).

Key things to know:
- In terms of efficacy, they are all about equal with the possible exception of clozapine, which seems to be better for the treatment of refractory cases of schizophrenia.
- The choice of drug relates to the side-effect profile, with the newer agents being favoured because of their lower rate of causing movement disorders.
- Side effects must be closely monitored, especially obesity, diabetes, hypertension and dyslipidaemia.
- Clozapine has the rare but potentially fatal side effect of agranulocytosis, and as a consequence, the patient must be on a blood monitoring system in

order to receive this medication. Cardiac monitoring is also required.

- The movement disorders (more common in treatment with the typicals) are called extrapyramidal side effects (EPSE), and are:
    - Acute dystonia (muscle stiffness that can be life-threatening if of the larynx)
    - Parkinsonism
    - Akathisia (a sort of restlessness)
    - Tardive dyskinesia (a delayed-onset movement problem that is very serious because it is sometimes irreversible).

    All of these have treatments, and sometimes the treatments are started at the time of the antipsychotic to prevent onset in high-risk people.

- A rare but potentially fatal side effect to be aware of is neuroleptic malignant syndrome (NMS), which causes fever, muscle stiffness, hypertension and confusion. If this occurs, hospital admission and emergency treatment are required.

- Some antipsychotics can be given by injection. The injections can be with a short-acting drug or long-acting drug (up to a month), which are called 'depot' injections. These are useful when adherence is problematic.

ANTI-ANXIETY MEDICATIONS

These are also called anxiolytics, and most are benzodiazepines.

Major uses: anxiety disorders (mainly generalised anxiety disorder and panic disorder), insomnia and many non-psychiatric related disorders such as epilepsy. Sometimes used for agitation, especially in severe depression or when first starting antidepressants.

Common examples: diazepam, clonazepam, oxazepam, temazepam, alprazolam.

Key things to know:
- The benzodiazepines are a group of medications with similar actions (sedative, anxiolytic, anticonvulsant and muscle relaxant) that have varying half-lives and are used for a broad range of disorders. They all have the potential for dependence.
- Treatment should aim to be short term.
- Some are predominantly used for insomnia (temazepam, flunitrazepam, nitrazepam) and others for anxiety (alprazolam, diazepam).
- None should be used without first warning the patient of potential dependence, especially with long-term use and increasing doses.
- Patients must be warned of the risks of driving or operating machinery while under the influence of benzodiazepines.

MOOD STABILISER MEDICATIONS

Major uses: bipolar disorder (for prophylaxis of episodes and acute treatment of mania and depression), augmentation of antidepressants when the depression is refractory, augmentation of antipsychotics when schizophrenia is refractory.

Common examples: lithium, carbamazepine, sodium valproate.

Key things to know:
- These are a complex group of drugs with complex side-effect profiles; mainly used in bipolar disorder.

- Each drug must be taken long term, and so careful monitoring of side effects is required.
- Lithium requires regular monitoring of plasma concentration as too low a level is non-therapeutic and too high is toxic. Lithium also affects thyroid and renal function so regular testing is required.
- There are major issues in taking these drugs during pregnancy and breastfeeding.

13

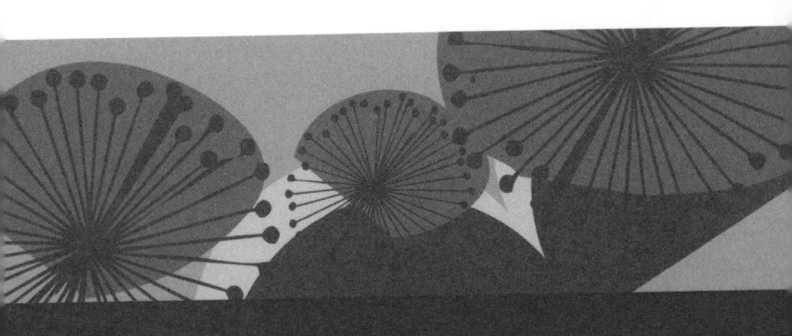

Psychotherapies

Psychotherapy = talking therapy. Pretty simple, isn't it? When people talk about psychotherapy they mean that someone is talking to someone else so that one of them (the patient, hopefully) feels better. Colloquially, psychotherapy has come to mean psychoanalysis (the stereotype is lying on the couch talking about your childhood). But really, psychotherapy means any type of talking that is therapeutic.

TYPES OF PSYCHOTHERAPY

While we'll be describing three types of psychotherapy there are in fact dozens. All types can be placed on a continuum. At one end of the continuum the patient does almost all the talking, at the other end the therapist does most of the talking. The former is called expressive psychotherapy and the latter, directive psychotherapy (see Figure 13.1).

BEHAVIOUR THERAPY

Behaviour therapy (BT) is where the patient is *directed* to do something. Fundamental to BT are *exposure* and *relaxation training*. For example, a patient with agoraphobia is exposed

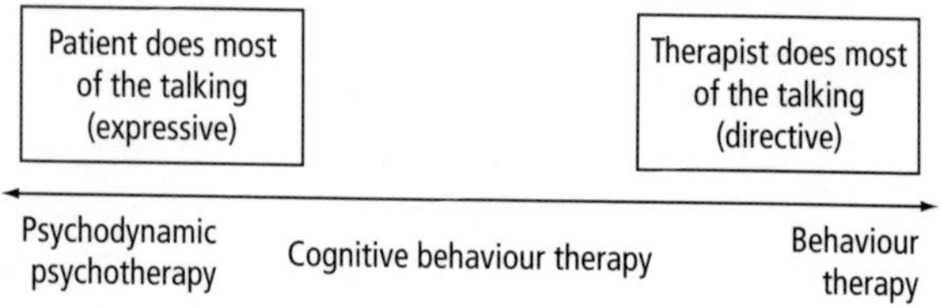

FIGURE 13.1 Psychotherapy continuum

to (real or imagined) increasing distances away from home after having performed relaxation training. This breaks the connection between being away from home and panic attacks. Another, basic, example is instructing the child patient to use the toilet just prior to sleeping (for enuresis). BT is very useful in the treatment of anxiety as well as other psychiatric disorders.

COGNITIVE BEHAVIOUR THERAPY

Cognitive behaviour therapy is currently the popular 'flavour' of psychotherapy. It combines BT with cognitive therapy (CT). Part of CT theory is that thoughts lead to feelings which lead to behaviours. If thoughts can be altered then so can the feelings and then the behaviours which will impact on the thoughts, and so on. For example, Lisa has the thought that she is unattractive and unpopular. That thought makes her feel sad. When her friend calls to ask her to a party on Saturday she says she's too down to go. Spending Saturday night alone makes Lisa think she doesn't have a social life so she feels sad, and so on.

CT employs the concept of *automatic thoughts* (as in the example above). These are the unhelpful, negative thoughts that pop up and make you feel sad or anxious. Very often they are irrational and have little evidence in reality. In CBT the therapist helps the patient identify these thoughts and then challenge them, as well as using behavioural strategies. The patient also learns how to problem solve. Along the way they must do homework (such as keeping a diary) and set goals.

CBT is useful for many psychiatric disorders but especially for depression and anxiety disorders. For CBT to be successful, patients must have a degree of psychological mindedness and a desire and commitment to change.

PSYCHODYNAMIC PSYCHOTHERAPY

Psychodynamic psychotherapy covers a range of expressive therapies. The underlying theory is that the parts of our unconscious and conscious are in a *dynamic* (or moving) flux. Also, feelings lead to thoughts which lead to behaviours. Most of our feelings come from unconscious impulses and drives developed during early childhood before we can put words to experiences, prior to forming *conscious* memories. In therapy, a key aim is to make the unconscious conscious so the associated emotional pain is lessened.

Psychodynamic psychotherapy is useful for many disorders, but especially for personality issues, mood disorders, adjustment disorders and relationship problems. As described in Chapter 10, for this form of therapy to be effective there are a number of advantageous patient characteristics.

The therapy can involve free association (talking about whatever comes into one's head), dreams (a rich vein of the unconscious, as are slips of the tongue or *Freudian slips*) and identifying transference. Transference is the collection of feelings the patient brings into the room that is unrelated to the therapist but are responses to events from some other time. For example, a woman with a long history of abuse by males immediately feels fearful of her new male therapist. Conversely, therapists have counter-transference which they must also monitor.

As part of the therapy process, the patient's (unconscious) *psychological defences* may be identified. The therapist may then discuss these with the patient in an effort to make the unconscious conscious. These defences are often at play in a range of disorders and situations.

CHAPTER 13 Psychotherapies

An easy way to understand these unconscious psychological defences is by using 'Ego', the 'defences canine':

Denial Mary's treasured dog, Ego, died two weeks ago, yet she still puts out his dinner every night.

Repression Jack loves the new puppy he bought but his wife Jane hates dogs. After three weeks Jane still can't remember Ego's name.

Displacement Barry had a hard day at work so he comes home and kicks the poor, innocent dog.

Intellectualisation Diane's beloved dog Ego is having an operation next week. Diane's friends are amazed at how 'well' she is coping. She unemotionally describes the operation in minute detail and the pathology of the tumour to be removed.

Rationalisation Paul desperately wants a dog but his wife won't allow him one because she just doesn't like dogs. Rather than feel angry with his wife he adopts her reasons for not getting a dog.

Humour After Ego died, Jack tells stories to his friends about how Ego used to poo on his angry neighbour's front lawn.

Projection Harry desperately wants to be a competitive runner but since breaking his leg he can't train. However, he now encourages his dog Ego to do laps around the park where he used to train.

Reaction formation Janine love her old family dog, Ego, but whenever she sees him she says, 'You know we ought to get rid of you, Ego, you're old and lazy'.

Acting out Bobby's parents favour his sister over him. Bobby takes the family dog and hides him in the garage. When asked why he did it he answers honestly that he doesn't know why.

14

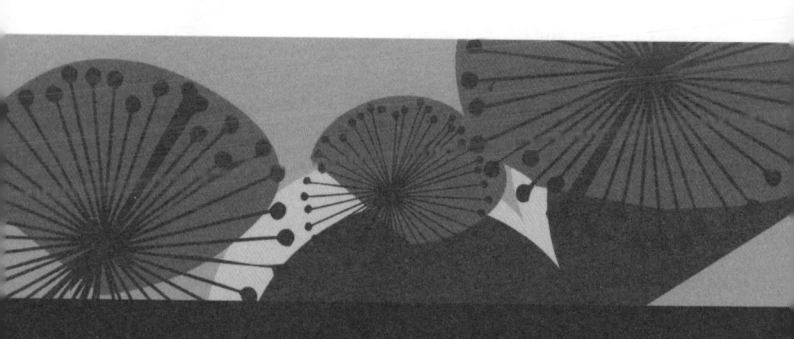

Child and adolescent psychiatry

Children grow up. Pretty basic fact. What you'll need to understand though is that they don't just grow up physically. They grow up cognitively (the capacity to think), emotionally, socially, motorically (find and gross motor) and in their use of language. At each age there are developmentally appropriate norms. These norms are helpful in guiding clinicians as to when children are having problems and also how to assess them. For example, speaking only in two-word sentences may be normal for a two year old but is out of the norm for a six year old.

ASSESSING THE CHILD

In child and adolescent psychiatry (CAP) the child or adolescent is called the *identified* patient. They are called this because while they may be the one with the presenting symptom, that symptom can sometimes be a reflection of the distress the family is undergoing. Children can often somatise their emotional distress. For example, consider a ten-year-old girl presenting with recurrent abdominal pain with no organic cause found, who is in the midst of a custody dispute, or a baby failing to thrive of a severely depressed mother. In these examples, you can see that the young patient is a barometer (an indicator) of their environment.

Assessing children and adolescents can be tricky. First of all, the child or adolescent must trust the clinician enough to allow them into their world. The patient may feel embarrassed or ashamed of their feelings or actions or those of others impacting on them. Gaining trust can take time, especially so if they have had negative experiences with adults ('why should I trust this one?').

Secondly, even though the child or adolescent may be very distressed they may not have the developmental skills to express their distress (feelings) in words. Imagine a three year old of a severely depressed parent – they wouldn't have the equivalent skills to verbalise their feelings (nor comment on those of their parents) as well as, say, a 14 year old. The developmental stage will thus determine the manner in which the internal world of the child is assessed. In young children this may be through watching their play or drawings.

Thirdly, the factors that contribute to disorders in children and adolescents can be complex and come from many sources. For example, a ten-year-old recent immigrant who presents with disruptive behaviour may be being bullied at school, have parents who must work long hours (and are thus unavailable), have a language difficulty (making reading in class both frustrating and boring) and have poor peer role models. Each one of these factors contributes to his presenting 'symptom'. Thus in CAP there is often a need to gain information from many sources. Teachers, parents, siblings, the GP and others can provide valuable information. For the same reasons, the multidisciplinary team is essential in the assessment to reach a diagnosis and formulation. Occupational therapists, speech therapists, psychologists, social workers, nurse practitioners and other disciplines (e.g. a cultural liaison worker) join with the psychiatrist to contribute to the assessment process.

Given these reasons, the assessment of a child or adolescent is rarely completed in one session. Many sessions may be needed. These include a family session, the child or adolescent alone and the parents alone. Different kinds of information can be gleaned from each. For example, the family's emotional tone (e.g. critical, light hearted, distant, warm, etc.) is important to note. In an individual session an adolescent may feel freer to speak his or her mind with the parents out of earshot, and visa versa.

Moreover, ensuing therapeutic sessions can add to the assessment picture. One of the keys in CAP is to keep an open mind to a change in the diagnosis/formulation. *Premature closure* (coming to a conclusion before all the facts are in) is an anathema.

TREATMENT

Treatment in CAP draws strongly on the bio-psycho-social paradigm. Because children and adolescents are mostly in the care of adults it is useful to engage those adults who contribute to that environment. Parents or carers and teachers are key to the management process.

Much of the management in CAP is through psychotherapies. Depending on the diagnosis, developmental stage and level of engagement, different psychotherapies are used. For example, behaviour therapy may be useful for a seven year old with nocturnal enuresis (e.g. a bell and pad). Parent therapy may help for a five year old with oppositional defiance disorder. Family therapy can be useful for an adolescent with an eating disorder. Classroom behaviour strategies (e.g. placing the child at the front desk) may be useful for managing a child with attention deficit hyperactivity disorder (ADHD). Cognitive behaviour therapy may be useful for a teenager with depression. Importantly, it is often not just one form of therapy that is used on one recipient. For example, a 16-year-old boy with depression could receive CBT individually, and he and his family could receive family therapy.

Biological therapies are used less as the primary treatment in CAP as compared to adult psychiatry. For example, antidepressants are generally not first line for treating adolescent depression. Antipsychotic medications are used as part of a broad range of psychosocial strategies for first-episode psychosis. One group of medications that is used more often in CAP than in adult psychiatry is the stimulants (e.g. methyl phenidate) for ADHD. It sounds counterintuitive but here stimulants actually help the patient to focus and settle.

SUMMARY

In summary, children and adolescents are always understood in the context of their families or carers, development and culture. Thus the care of their condition will incorporate these contexts into the treatment plan. Some of the conditions seen in CAP that you should become familiar with are:

- Oppositional defiant disorder
- Autism spectrum disorders
- Eating disorders
- First-episode psychosis
- Attention deficit hyperactivity disorder
- Conduct disorders
- Adolescent depression
- Anxiety disorders.

15

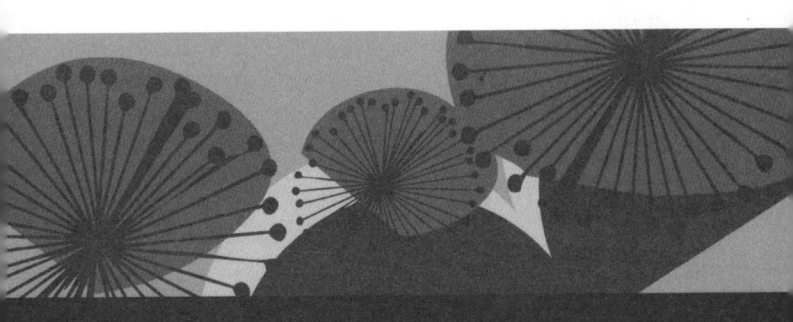

Old age psychiatry

People are living longer and having fewer children. As a consequence our population is ageing. By current trends, 25 per cent of our population will be over 65 by 2050. Ageing poses a range of challenges to mental health, from the ageing brain to the losses of growing old, such as the death of loved ones, the loss of independence and the loss of physical health.

TYPES OF DISORDERS

The most common psychiatric disorders of old age are depressive disorders, cognitive disorders (especially dementia and delirium), anxiety disorders (especially phobias) and alcohol-related disorders.

ASSESSING ELDERLY PATIENTS

Assessment of the elderly requires some special skills, such as the ability to perform a good cognitive assessment, but even more importantly, it requires you to be particularly good at your job! The history is longer (older patients generally have had more illness episodes), it is harder to take (because of difficulties such as poor hearing), the information is sometimes less reliable (due to cognitive impairment), and integrating all the information and untangling the medical comorbidity requires a lot of skill.

On top of the usual history and examination, there are three things you must not forget (the three Cs of assessing elderly patients): you must obtain *collateral* history, you must do a *cognitive* assessment, and you must explore *comorbid* medical problems.

Collateral information is information you learn from sources other than the patient—typically the family or the general practitioner. This gives you the baseline state of the patient and the rate of decline. In any cognitive disorder, this is particularly important, as the timeline is the main clue to the diagnosis.

Cognition, in its simplest form, just means thinking. Cognitive assessment means assessing the various tasks that go into thinking, such as orientation, attention, language and memory. Simple cognitive testing usually assesses whether the patient is alert and oriented and how their short-term memory is working. A detailed cognitive assessment, usually performed by a neuropsychologist, takes a couple of hours and includes all of the above plus intelligence, visuospacial skills, constructional ability, mathematics and various 'executive functions' like planning and judgment.

The mini-mental state examination (MMSE) is by far the most used structured, bedside cognitive test. The MMSE covers orientation, memory, attention, calculation, language and the ability to follow simple commands. It is scored out of 30, and as a rough rule of thumb a score below 25 *suggests* impairment (so more detailed testing is required). It is routinely performed on admission for elderly patients, and serial (or repeated) testing is used to monitor progress. Learn it; you will do it many, many times between now and your own old age.

DEMENTIA

Dementia is a gradual onset of global impairment in cognitive functioning in the absence of impaired consciousness (i.e. in the absence of delirium). The prevalence is 1 per cent at age

65, and then doubles every five years. It can also occur in younger adults but is rare.

There are a number of different types of dementia. Each starts in its own characteristic way, but they each eventually become global, affecting all cognitive functions. The commonest forms are Alzheimer's disease (about 50 per cent), vascular (about 15 per cent), Lewy Body (about 15 per cent), and then the various mixed forms. Less common causes include Parkinson's disease, Huntington disease, HIV-related, alcohol-related and head-trauma-related dementia.

Distinguishing between the various dementias can be a real challenge, as the clinical course, associated symptoms and investigations can overlap, especially in the early stages. Determining the type of dementia definitively must sometimes wait until post mortem.

The management of dementia involves many of the health professions and depends on the stage of the dementia. There are medications to treat the actual dementia (such as acetylcholinesterase inhibitors in Alzheimer's disease) and medications that help with associated symptoms (such as antipsychotics for hallucinations), but most of the treatment is more psychosocial. Optimising independent living, managing behavioural disturbance and supporting the family and carers are some of the keys to a successful management plan.

DELIRIUM

Delirium is an acute onset of fluctuating cognitive impairment and consciousness. Any acute onset, fluctuating change in mental state is a delirium until proved otherwise, and it's time to do a thorough physical examination and get your pad and pen to start ordering a few tests! It's a syndrome with many possible causes, and is commonly seen in the hospital setting. The causes can be summarised with the mnemonic DELIRIUM—**D**rugs, **E**ndocrine, **L**ung (anything that causes hypoxia), **I**nfections, **R**enal, **I**schaemia (like strokes, infarcted bowel or heart), **U**nknown (this is the commonest! No cause is identified in about 30 per cent of cases) and **M**etabolic.

Delirium can present in the community and needs to be distinguished from dementia, which can be hard if you don't know the patient (hence the importance of collateral history). Delirium is one of the commonest referrals to the consultation-liaison psychiatry service. There are two good reasons for this. Firstly, it is often confused with psychosis (a third of delirious patients have psychotic symptoms) so the psychiatrist is called in to assess the mental state. Secondly, delirious patients are often behaviourally disturbed—they shout out, get paranoid, wander, are awake at night and sometimes hit out at staff that they mistakenly think are attacking them. To improve this we use a combination of environmental changes and medications. The environmental changes include a quiet room with steady lighting, and reorientation cues such as the day and date on the wall, the name of the hospital and photos of loved ones. Being delirious is like constantly waking from a bad dream, so you have to constantly reorientate the patient as they go in and out of consciousness.

Medications used include sedatives to aid night-time sleep and antipsychotics to treat psychotic symptoms. The challenge here is to use the bare minimum dose, because sedating medications may worsen the delirium.

Index

A

abnormality
    distinguishing from normality, 2–3
abuse *see* drug abuse
adolescents *see* child and adolescent psychology
affect (clue in MSEs), 14
alcohol, 48–9
    see also drug and alcohol disorders
amphetamines, 49
anti-anxiety medications, 66–7
antidepressant medications, 64–5
antipsychotic medications, 65–6
anxiety disorders, 9, 41–5
    treatment, 44–5
appearance (clue in MSEs), 13
assessments
    interviews, 8–11
    old age psychology, 80–1
    risk management, 26–8
attenuation of stressors, 27–8

B

behaviour (clue in MSEs), 13
behaviour therapy, 70–3
bipolar disorder, 10, 32
    treatment, 33–4
borderline personality disorder (BPD), 54–6
    aetiology, 55–6
    treatment, 56
BPD *see* borderline personality disorder

C

C-L psychiatry *see* consultation-liaison psychiatry
cannabis, 49
CAP *see* child and adolescent psychology
catatonia, 37
CHAIR, 25–6
child and adolescent psychology (CAP), 75–8
    assessment, 75–7
    biological therapies, 78
    treatment, 77–8
circumstantiality (clue in MSEs), 16
classification
    personality disorders, 54
    in psychiatry, 2
clothing (clue in MSEs), 13
cocaine, 50
cognition (clue in MSEs), 17
cognitive behaviour therapy, 71
command hallucinations, 37
consultation-liaison
    psychiatry, 58–61
    role, 58
    special problems, 58–61
content (clue in MSEs), 16
conversion disorder, 60

D

delirium, elderly patients, 82–3
delusions, 37
dementia, 81–2
dependence, 48

Index

depression, 10, 30
    in the mentally ill, 58–9
    symptoms, 30–1
    treatment, 32–3
depressive episodes
    bipolar disorder, 33–4
derailment (clue in MSEs), 16
diagnostic hierarchy, 3–5
diagnostic manuals, 5
drug abuse, 48
drug and alcohol disorders, 47–51
drugs, 48–51
dysthymia, 31

E

ecstasy, 51
Ego (defences canine), 73
eye contact (clue in MSEs), 14

F

first episode psychosis (FEP), 37–8
flight of ideas (clue in MSEs), 16
follow up (risk management), 28
formal thought disorder (FTD), 15
formulations, 20
    case study, 20–1
    writing, 21–2
fraternity (risk management), 28
FTD *see* formal thought disorder

G

GAD *see* generalised anxiety disorder
generalised anxiety disorder (GAD), 10, 43

H

hallucinations, 37
histories, taking, 8–11

hygiene (clue in MSEs), 13
hypochondriasis, 60

I

insight (clue in MSEs), 17
interviews, 19
intoxication, 47

J

judgment, (clue in MSEs), 17

M

manic episodes
    bipolar disorder, 34
medications, 63
    types, 63–8
mental state examinations (MSEs), 13–17
mood stabiliser medications, 67–8
movements (clue in MSEs), 14
MSEs *see* mental state examinations

N

normality
    distinguishing from abnormality, 2–3

O

obsessive compulsive disorder (OCD), 9, 42–3
old age psychology, 80–3
    assessment, 80–1
    types of disorders, 80
opioids, 50

P

panic disorder, 10, 41–2
paraphrenia, 36
pathological anxiety, 43

patient histories *see* histories
perception (clue in MSEs), 17
perserveration (clue in MSEs), 16
personality
　defined, 53
　development, 53–4
personality disorders, 53–6
　classification, 54
treatment, 56
phobias, 42
post-traumatic stress disorder, 10, 43
posture (clue in MSEs), 14
primary anxiety vs secondary anxiety, 44
psychodynamic psychotherapy, 72–3
psychosis, 10, 36
psychotherapy, 70
　types, 70–3

R

rapport, (clue in MSEs), 17
risk assessments
　process, 25–6
　purpose, 24–5
risk factors, 26
risk management, 26–8

S

safety (risk management), 27
schizophrenia, 36
　diagnosis, 36–9
　management, 39
medication, 39
secondary anxiety vs primary anxiety, 44
social anxiety disorder, 10, 42
somatisation disorder, 61
somatoform disorders, 60–1
speech (clue in MSEs), 14
STAFF (risk management technique), 26–8
stressors, attenuation, 27–8
symptoms, 4
　timeline, 5
syndromes, 3

T

tangentiality (clue in MSEs), 16
thought (clue in MSEs), 15
treatment (risk management), 27

W

withdrawal, 47–8